Evidence-Based Medicine on the Trail

Evidence-Based Medicine on the Trail

A CASE STUDY APPROACH

First Edition

R. David Doan III, MS, PA-C
Western Michigan University

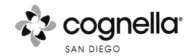

cognella®
SAN DIEGO

Bassim Hamadeh, CEO and Publisher
Jennifer Codner, Senior Field Acquisitions Editor
Susana Christie, Senior Developmental Editor
Michelle Piehl, Senior Project Editor
Abbey Hastings, Production Editor
Asfa Arshi, Graphic Design Assistant
Trey Soto, Licensing Specialist
Kim Scott/Bumpy Design, Interior Designer
Natalie Piccotti, Director of Marketing
Kassie Graves, Senior Vice President, Editorial
Jamie Giganti, Director of Academic Publishing

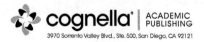

cognella® | ACADEMIC PUBLISHING
3970 Sorrento Valley Blvd., Ste. 500, San Diego, CA 92121

*To the Western Michigan University Physician Assistant class of 2020,
thank you for being my guinea pigs and for all your support.*

*To the class of 2021, thank you for embracing the story and cases and for
adapting to virtual lessons during the COVID-19 pandemic. Your optimism
and enthusiasm are awe-inspiring and infectious ... in a good way.*

Table of Contents

Patient Files

Preface

Evidence-Based Medicine on the Trail is not your typical textbook. A quick glance at the chapters found in the table of contents might cause you to wonder if you picked up the wrong book. I assure you, you did not. This book was written and designed with real-world practice in mind. It is intended to provide real-world patient scenarios for students to examine and use as a basis for asking clinical questions, searching for answers, and critiquing their findings with an evidence-based medicine (EBM) approach. The setting of the story behind the cases is meant to provide an experience similar to that of a clinical rotation, while providing the occasional clinical pearl and entertainment along the way.

Instructors, how should you use this book? This book was intended to be completed after the basics of EBM have been taught. It was written for practicing previously learned EBM skills. The book is broken up into six "days" in the clinic, with each day designated by a different chapter. Each day, or chapter, has six case studies, with the exception of the last day/chapter, which has only three case studies. I would suggest using a day/chapter per lecture hour and assigning each case study in the chapters to small groups for study. A good group size could be anywhere up to six students. Each group would be charged with coming up with a good, researchable PICO question and then asked to go out and find the answer to their question using skills learned previously in their research/EBM classes. I have provided a sample appraisal sheet in the book's appendix that can be used to guide their critique of the information they find in answering research questions (several other options can be found with a simple online search). I would suggest they either present their case and findings to the class or provide a summary to you in a SOAP note and summary of research findings—your choice.

Students, how should *you* use this book? I've found the best way to learn is hands-on. We've all heard the phrase, "See one, do one, teach one," right? Examples in class that are done for you are fine for studying, but actually *doing* the work is the way you get comfortable in your skills. I've put together a number of clinical cases for you to sink your teeth into, with a wide variety of clinical scenarios, character types you may see in a clinic, and moral conundrums you may encounter. I would encourage you to ask as many questions as possible when encountering these patients. Ask background questions that you didn't have time to look up in your other classes. Ask foreground, or PICO, questions, and dig deeper in your understanding of the best evidence in each of their situations.

Pay attention to the characters for clinical pearls, and watch for sidebars that provide extra tidbits of knowledge in some of the cases as well.

It is my opinion that the best way to learn is to have fun while learning. I also find that students remember better what they've learned when the facts or information are coupled with a memorable case or patient. I hope you find these patients and cases memorable and useful in your attempt to master your EBM approach.

I would be remiss if I didn't say something about the setting and happenings in the story behind the cases. Munising and Christmas are actual cities in the Upper Peninsula of Michigan (U.P.). The area is absolutely breathtaking, and I encourage you all to visit if given the chance. The trails are real, the island is real, and it is *almost* all real. The clinic in the story doesn't exist, and if you searched for it on Google Earth, you'd likely find an empty sand lot. The people in the story are also fictitious, despite their believable characteristics or any similarities in names (none intended, I promise). The negative aspects of some of the story characters should by no means reflect any of the wonderful people who live and work in the U.P. As far as I know, there are no nefarious activities going on in the Munising area, and the people who live and work there have been fabulous in all my experiences.

Lastly, this book is a tribute to all of you! I have worked with physician assistant students for many years and have loved every moment. Thank you for picking up my labor of love—enjoy the ride!

Welcome to the U.P.

Charlie Brinker was excited to finally start his last clinical rotation for PA school. He was extra excited to be having his rotation in the Upper Peninsula of Michigan (U.P.) through June and July. He loved camping, hiking, fishing, and doing anything outdoors, so ending his year of rotations on the shores of Lake Superior was extra special. The rotation was at an urgent care clinic that acted more like a family practice office to locals and tourists who lived or visited the area near Munising, Michigan. It was managed by a physician assistant (PA) named Dave Harrington who loved teaching PA students and was rumored to teach them more about life than just medicine. He was a favorite among the students who rotated with him, and Charlie couldn't have been more ready to meet him.

Although there were options for lodging in the neighboring town of Christmas, Charlie opted to set up camp in the campground next to the clinic. He arrived the Friday before his rotation was set to begin and got a nice spot by the lake. The campground was nearly empty as the tourism season was just starting. He was only a quarter mile walk to the clinic and near the Pipeline trailhead that was located across the street from the campground. The weather was cool and spring-like, but he didn't mind. He was really looking forward to spending the next two months living by the lake and enjoying himself on the trails (and learning, of course). He expected a relaxing atmosphere; he never would have guessed that he would find himself in the middle of so much drama in the quiet U.P.

* * *

Dave Harrington arrived at the clinic just before 9 a.m., still a good hour before office hours. Dawn, the clinic's newly hired nurse who also served as the receptionist, wouldn't be in until 9:30 a.m. He was expecting a PA student this morning to start a two-month rotation. The student was advised to show up before 10 a.m., the start of the schedule. Dave liked to arrive early and sit alone on the back patio to look out across the bay to Grand Island. This morning he breathed in the scent of fish and pine in the air. It was cool and sunny, as summer was reluctant to take over spring. June marked the unofficial start of the summer tourism season in the small town of Christmas. Better known for the winter season associated with the city's name (you can't seem to avoid a Santa or Mrs. Claus in a storefront or on a sign in this town), Christmas was also a draw for nature lovers and gamblers during the U.P. summers. The neighboring town of Munising, only about three miles down the road, offered boat tours to view the many shipwrecks in the bay area and to see the splendor of Pictured Rocks National Lakeshore Park along the southern shores of Lake Superior. The clinic sat along the lakeshore on M-28, nestled next to a campground and only about a mile from the town of Christmas and the Kewadin Casino. The clinic opened every June and closed at the end of every September, mirroring the tourism season.

Dave had moved to Michigan's Upper Peninsula about six years earlier, planning to get away from the busy clinics downstate and get into nature. He immediately found the laid-back lifestyle of yooper life and the serenity of his surroundings to his liking. He had even been known to camp in the backcountry for weeks and hike back and forth from the office. During the "off-season" he worked at Marquette General as a general surgery PA, but in the summers, he preferred working at Tourist Park Urgent Care Center. He was the sole provider at the clinic that was owned by Dr. Robertson, a physician in Marquette. He worked alone to evaluate the patients there. Dr. Roberson had a collaborative agreement with Dave, much like a supervising physician in other states.

On most days Dave saw only a handful of patients, usually for ailments related to camping or hiking mishaps. Occasionally he would see a tourist from Christmas—mostly gamblers from the Kewadin Casino—or a few locals—friends of his or folks who couldn't get into their regular provider and didn't want to head into town. But most of his patients were tourists here for the hiking or backcountry camping. The big draw was the North Country Trail and its many offshoots in the area. The U.P. is home to Pictured Rocks National Lakeshore and close to twenty state parks that make up 3.8 million acres of land, so naturally, campers and hikers frequented the area around the clinic. Business was usually pretty slow in June as the season kicked off, but by August, he would be busy as the parks and trails filled to capacity.

CHAPTER 1

Monday

At 9:30 a.m. sharp—it's always important to be punctual on your first day of a rotation—Charlie Brinker arrived at the office as Dawn was unlocking the front door. She gave him a quick tour and then unlocked the back door so Dave could come in from the patio where he waited. As 10 a.m. approached, Dave, Dawn, and Charlie made sure the shelves were stocked and the office was ready to receive patients. They didn't expect to be too busy on the first day of the season, but Dave liked to teach each incoming student the importance of being a team player. He stressed, "Every person in the clinic is on the same team and should work together to care for our patients. No one player is more important or above helping where needed." With the preparations done, Dave and Charlie sat on the back patio to drink coffee, discuss expectations for the rotation, and get to know each other better.

Dawn poked her head through the door to let them know that there was someone at the front desk.

"Joseph Murphy is here to see ya."

"Just to say hello? Or does he need to be seen?" Dave asked.

"Both, I'd guess," she replied.

"Well, all right. Get him into a room, and I'll be right there."

Dave got up, set down his coffee mug, and headed in to grab his stethoscope and clipboard. Charlie scrambled to follow. He'd be shadowing Dave today. He was instructed to jot down questions and look them up for research at the end of the day. The following day he would have to give a report to Dave.

Joseph was Dave's oldest friend in the U.P. They met soon after Dave moved to Christmas. They were both hiking through the backcountry on seldom-used trails between the Pipeline trail and Old Golf Course Road. Dave had been resting on a log when Joseph came along. They sparked up a conversation about the woods, talked hiking and camping, and found they had a lot in common. Both were avid hikers and considered themselves naturalists, meaning they enjoyed studying nature. Dave's love for nature stemmed from his days in the Boy Scouts, while Joseph came by his love for nature naturally as a native born in the Sault Ste. Marie Tribe of Chippewas who had been taught to respect and love nature.

1

Over the years, they had met on the trails to discuss their findings and methods to improve the conditions along the trails. They founded their friendship on mutual respect and trust, so naturally, when Joseph was diagnosed with diabetes, he placed his trust in Dave to walk him through treatment. Joseph told Dave he had been diagnosed by the tribal clinic provider, but he hadn't gotten education about it from the tribe. He asked if Dave knew anything about diabetes and was astonished to learn that Dave was a physician assistant. From then on, Joseph referred to him as Doc, regardless of how many times Dave tried to correct him. Although Dave only worked four months out of the year in this part of the U.P., Joseph valued his opinion above that of all other medical professionals. He soon started seeing Dave at least once each summer in the clinic for his diabetes, and of course whenever he had any other medical question.

• • •

Joseph R. Murphy and the Question of Insulin Management
Monday, June 1
10:15 AM
Patient: Joseph R. Murphy
Age: 42

As they entered the patient room (one of only three in the small office), Joseph stood and took two large strides across the room to give Dave a bear hug. Joseph was a large man, standing six feet three inches and weighing around 230 pounds. Dave appeared to momentarily lose his breath. Joseph released him from his embrace, took a step back, and held Dave's shoulders out in front of him to give him a once-over.

"You're too skinny, Doc!" he said, giving a playful light backhand to Dave's midsection. "They forget to feed you up there in Marquette? You look like a starved deer! You need to eat some of my wife's cooking!"

"I'm pretty sure Mary's cooking is what caused your diabetes. No thanks," he replied with a chuckle. He sat down at the counter and gestured for Joseph to sit as well. "So, what brings you in today? I usually don't see you for your diabetes visit for a couple more weeks. Everything all right?"

"What? Can't a guy just come in to see his buddy on the first day of the season? Who says there's gotta be something wrong? I just wanted to say 'hi' and wish you luck this season." Joseph looked to the door and saw Charlie standing there. "Who's this?"

"This here is Charlie Brinker. He's a PA student who'll be with me for the next two months," Dave replied.

"You listen to this man. He's smarter than he looks!" Joseph said with a hearty chuckle. "Well, since you are my doc and all, and you know I trust only you with my health, I gotta be honest with you, Doc. I haven't been taking my insulin this month."

"Why not?"

"Well, because you weren't around in the off-season, I went to the tribal clinic a few months ago. They changed my meds up a little. Gave me some new insulin that I don't think is working as well."

"Joe, you can't just stop taking insulin. It's not safe!"

Joseph reached down and grabbed his backpack off the floor and started rummaging through it until he found what he was looking for. He handed Dave a small box. Dave recognized it instantly.

"This is mixed 70/30 insulin. What happened to the long-acting and short-acting insulins that I gave you?"

Joseph shrugged. "They gave me that because it was cheaper than the stuff you gave me. Said I only had to do two shots now instead of four. Sounded good to me, but my sugars ain't been so great."

"I'm not a fan of mixed insulin. I'd rather you take your insulin basal/bolus like I taught you last fall."

"You know I'll do whatever you say, Doc. Just say the word."

"I'll get you a new script, but don't ever just stop taking your insulin. You have a question, you call me first before you do something like this again. I'm serious!" Dave handed the new prescription to Joseph. "Now, Dawn said you had something for me?" Dave asked, while jotting down the instructions for the new insulin regimen on a separate piece of paper.

With a big grin, Joseph reached back into his backpack. "Sure do, Doc!" He reached in and pulled out a shoebox. Beaming with pride, he handed it over to Dave. "A gift to start your season out right!"

Dave took the box and opened it. Inside was a knife with a roughly five-inch blade and an antler handle in a leather sheath. Etched in the handle was the word "DOC," and the leather sheath was decorated with fine leatherwork featuring the region's animals and plants.

"Wow, Joe. This is wonderful. Did you do this?"

"Nope, I had it made for you. I got a job now," he replied, puffing his chest out and smiling.

"Now that's some interesting news! Who in their right mind decided you'd be a good hire?" Dave asked with a chuckle.

"I'm working security at the Kewadin Casino. Mostly with the money transfers. They probably thought because I know the woods so well, I'd be a good guy to have."

"That's great, Joe! Now you can pay me back for all those IOUs!" Dave said with a laugh. "No, really, I'm glad you found some work. Does that mean I won't see you on the trails this summer?"

"Well, you might still see me once in a while. I'll be escorting the money to the airfield, and I know you hike out that ways some days. Can't get rid of me that easily, heh?"

"I guess not. I'm sure we'll bump into each other; we usually do. Now take that script to the pharmacy and get started on that insulin!"

"You got it, Doc. You're the boss."

• • •

When Joseph left, Dave and Charlie returned to the patio table and refreshed their coffees. Dave asked Charlie questions, quizzing him on his knowledge of diabetic management. Charlie realized that he had some questions about insulin therapy. Specifically, he had come up with a foreground (PICO) question about insulins:

"When treating type 2 diabetics with insulin, does use of a mixed insulin work as effectively as using the basal/bolus method in lowering hemoglobin A1c?"

ASSIGNMENT

Help Charlie research his foreground (PICO) question. Find a study that answers Charlie's question, and appraise it for its Validity, Importance, and Usefulness. You can use the worksheet found in the appendix as a guide.

Next, write a brief summary of the study, why you feel it answers Charlie's question adequately, and whether the study was valid, important, and useful in this case. What are some of the pros and cons of the study, and how will it impact Joseph's care? What would you do for Joseph after researching this question if you were the PA caring for him?

• • •

Terry J. Lautner and the Case of Foot Pain

Monday, June 1

11:00 AM

Patient: Terry J. Lautner

Age: 47

Later that morning, Dave and Charlie entered room two together to see their next patient. Charlie was advised to do all the talking, while Dave observed. He'd fill in the gaps if he felt questions were overlooked. They were seeing Terry Lautner, who told Dawn he was having severe toe and foot pain.

"Good morning, Mr. Lautner, my name's Charlie, and I'm a PA student working with Mr. Harrington today."

Dave gave a quick wave from behind Charlie.

Charlie took the seat at the small table against the wall and faced Terry while Dave leaned against the closed door.

"What brings you in the office today?" Charlie asked.

"My left foot is killing me. It started hurting a little yesterday afternoon and got worse throughout the evening. This morning when I got up, the pain was unbearable. I can't even walk without pain. I tried ibuprofen, but it didn't seem to help much. I tried using ice too. Nothing seems to help!"

"What were you doing yesterday before it started hurting? Did you injure the foot somehow?" Charlie asked.

"I was riding my bike on some trails yesterday. There's some awesome trails around here if you like trail riding. I don't think I injured it though. I mean, I'd know if I got hurt, wouldn't I?" Terry replied.

"Where is the pain? Can you describe the pain?" Charlie asked.

"It hurts on the middle of the foot, kind of on the side, I guess. It aches all the time, and it's worse when I put weight on it or even when it touches anything. Wearing a shoe is torture," Terry replied with a grimace.

"On a scale from zero to ten, with ten being the worst pain you've ever felt, how would you rate your pain?" Charlie asked.

"It's like a six or seven most of the time, but when I get up to walk, it's a nine. I had a kidney stone last summer. Now that was a ten. This is bad, just not kidney-stone bad."

Charlie looked a little puzzled, and then he asked, "Is there any pain on the heel of the foot?" He thought maybe Terry had plantar fasciitis.

"No. Like I said, it's on the top of the foot and on the outside of the foot in the middle."

Charlie looked to Dave for guidance. Dave walked toward Terry and had him lift up his foot for examination. It looked a little swollen, but wasn't erythematous.

"You said it hurts to touch?" Dave asked.

"Yeah, just having my shoe on makes it hurt," Terry said.

"Do you drink much beer?" Dave asked.

"What does that have to do with anything?" Terry replied defensively.

"Well, if you've been drinking more beer lately, you could be dealing with a gout flare-up in your foot. That could be pretty painful. Did you drink beer recently?" Dave asked.

Terry sighed. "I always get a drink at the Legion after my shift at the casino. I might've had a few more beers last night than usual. You really think beer did this?" Terry asked, as he lifted his foot for emphasis. "I don't really want to give up beer, doc."

Regular alcohol consumption, whether it is beer, spirits, or wine, can increase risk for gout flares. Even patients who are considered low-risk or moderate consumers of alcohol (one to two drinks per day) should be advised to reduce their consumption of alcohol to help prevent future gout flares (Choi et al. 2004).

"Well, I certainly think it's gout; we'll get some labs to confirm. In the mean-time, we'll fix you up with some medication and get you feeling better."

• • •

Dave and Charlie exited the room to discuss diagnosis and treatment of gout. They discussed the role of diet and alcohol in relation to gout. Dave asked Charlie to look into some of these areas and report back the next day with what he found.

ASSIGNMENT

Come up with a foreground (PICO) question based on this case. Find a study that answers your question, and appraise it for its Validity, Impor-tance, and Usefulness. Use the worksheet in the appendix, and write a brief summary of the study, why you feel it answers your question ade-quately, and whether the study was valid, important, and useful in this case. What are some of the pros and cons of the study, and how will it impact the patient's care? What would you do after researching this question if you were the PA caring for this patient?

• • •

Jason K. Varney and the Question on Burn Care

Monday, June 1

11:30 AM

Patient: Jason K. Varney

Age: 37

Charlie was sent into room three to get a history on their next patient, Jason K. Varney, who was at the clinic to have a burn evaluated.

"Good morning, Mr. Varney. My name is Charlie, and I'm a PA student working with Mr. Harrington. I hear you're here today to have a burn looked at?"

"That's me," Jason replied, waving his left hand briefly to point out the bandaged hand. "Burned it in a campfire. I immediately stuck it in the water bucket that was next to the fire. I put a layer of honey on it and wrapped it. Haven't looked at it since. That was three days ago. It took me that long to get here."

For the first day or two, burn wounds are fairly sterile, but they can colonize with bacteria soon after and lead to infection. Several agents can be prescribed to minimize bacterial counts. There are some nonprescription agents that have been used as well, such as aloe vera, honey, and sugar paste. Honey has been considered an ancient traditional remedy for wounds and has actually been found to be quite effective in inhibiting *Pseudomonas* (Bitter and Erickson 2016).

Charlie was confused and didn't understand what Jason meant by the time it took to get to the office.

Jason must have understood the perplexed look on Charlie's face because he clarified: "I was hiking the North Country Trail and had a reservation here in Munising at the campground next door. It was a long hike. I just got into camp this morning. After setting up camp here, I came right in. I knew honey was once used for burns, but I probably need antibiotics or something, right?"

"Well, I'll need to see the wound to know if you need antibiotics, but I have a few more questions I need to ask first. Are your vaccinations up-to-date?"

"I don't know. I mean, I'm sure I had all my shots as a kid, but I haven't had a shot in over a decade at least."

"Were there any chemicals in the fire? Like, did you use gas to start it or anything like that?"

"Nope. Just plain old matches and kindling."

Because he wasn't sure if honey would make things worse or not, Charlie asked about signs of infection. Jason's answers seemed to indicate that he was fairly healthy.

"Well, let's have a look at it," Charlie finally agreed.

Jason started slowly unraveling the gauze from around the burn on his left hand. Expecting to see a gruesome burn, Charlie was surprised to find that it didn't really look all that bad. Sure, the burn was extensive, but there was no pus or discharge other than a yellowish, slime-like film. Charlie thought this could be from the honey, not infection.

"Not too bad. I was expecting worse. Let me get Dave in here to look at it, and we'll get to fixing you up."

Back in the hallway, Charlie told Dave what he had learned from Jason, and together they reviewed care for burns. He would need a tetanus booster for sure, but Dave wanted to see the wound before making a judgment on the need for antibiotics.

They both returned to the room, and after a brief introduction, Dave took a look at the wound. The burn covered about eighty percent of the dorsum on Jason's left hand and wasn't too deep. The index and middle finger were also burned. The edges of the burn appeared to be ashen gray and peeling. The flesh in the center of the wound was red and raw looking. There was a yellow-gray film over most of the burn.

"By the pattern of the burn, it looks like you may have reached too close to the flame for something. Am I right?" asked Dave.

"I dropped something in the fire that I couldn't let burn. When I reached in and grabbed it, the wood in the fire shifted and hit my hand."

"Well, it looks like the honey did a fine job of keeping it from getting worse, but I'm sorry to say, you'll need a tetanus shot. I'll get you some topical silver sulfadiazine for the burn, and we'll have to debride the wound as well."

Dave showed Charlie the basics for wound debridement and let him finish. Because there was nothing else to do while he worked on the wound, Charlie passed the time by talking to Jason about his hiking. He learned that Jason was once in the Army and was now taking time in the woods to try and clear his head. He had been backpacking across the U.P. for the past six weeks. Before setting out on this hike, he had found it difficult to keep a job due to his PTSD. He had lost at a casino what little he had saved and now was living off the land and occasionally camping in campgrounds. He said he planned to stay at the Munising Tourist Park Campground for a few nights, but would have to camp in the backcountry soon due to his dwindling money. He'd have to use patient assistance to cover subsequent debridements, if he needed them.

When the burn was cleaned and treated, Charlie rewrapped the wound, and Dave gave Jason a prescription for the silver sulfadiazine, advised him to keep it clean, and told him to return in a few days.

· · ·

Out on the patio, Dave and Charlie discussed Jason's burn and subsequent treatment. Charlie again came up with some good clinical questions.

ASSIGNMENT

Come up with a foreground (PICO) question based on this case. Find a study that answers your question, and appraise it for its Validity, Importance, and Usefulness. Use the worksheet in the appendix, and write a brief summary of the study, why you feel it answers your question adequately, and whether the study was valid, important, and useful in this case. What are some of the pros and cons of the study, and how will it impact the patient's care? What would you do after researching this question if you were the PA caring for this patient?

· · ·

Becky W. Clay and the Case of Swimmer's Itch

Monday, June 1

1:30 PM

Patient: Becky W. Clay

Age: 12

After lunch, Dave sent Charlie in to see Becky Clay, who was in the clinic with her mother to have a rash looked at. When Charlie entered the exam room, he found Becky sitting on the exam table with her knees up to her chest. She was scratching excessively at her lower legs. Mrs. Clay was standing next to her and trying to get her to stop scratching.

Charlie set his clipboard on the table and reached out to shake Mrs. Clay's hand.

"Good afternoon, I'm Charlie. I'm a PA student working with Mr. Harrington today. If you don't mind, I'll be getting some info for Mr. Harrington before he sees Becky. Dawn tells us you're here with a rash you'd like to have looked at."

"That's right. Becky has been itching her ankles all morning. She has scratched herself silly. I mean, just look at her ankles. Some of her scratch marks have started to bleed!" Mrs. Clay said.

"Have you been itching them all morning Becky?" Charlie asked.

At Charlie's question Becky stopped itching and blushed. "No," she replied quietly.

"Yes, she has," Mrs. Clay remarked. "I think it was because we were looking for Yooperlites the last few nights along the beach. She was wading in some water pools by the beach that were just deeper than her ankles, and she's been itching her lower legs ever since."

Charlie stopped writing and looked up at Mrs. Clay.

"What are Yooperlites?"

"Oh, they're these rocks you can find along the Lake Superior shoreline that glow orange spots under a black light. You have to look for them at night. That's why we were out there the last few nights," Mrs. Clay explained.

"I see," Charlie said. "Do you think she could have walked through some poison ivy when you were by the beach?"

"No. There isn't any poison ivy around there. I think she's got swimmer's itch," Mrs. Clay said.

Charlie thought she might be right. It made sense. Swimmer's itch is caused by a parasite found in snails in lakes and ponds. They cause an allergic reaction when they burrow into the skin of an unsuspecting swimmer—or in this case, a Yooperlite hunter. He wasn't entirely sure what the best treatment for swimmer's itch was, so he told Becky and Mrs. Clay he would talk it over with Dave and they would come back in to talk about treatment options.

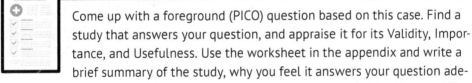

ASSIGNMENT

Come up with a foreground (PICO) question based on this case. Find a study that answers your question, and appraise it for its Validity, Importance, and Usefulness. Use the worksheet in the appendix and write a brief summary of the study, why you feel it answers your question adequately, and whether the study was valid, important, and useful in this case. What are some of the pros and cons of the study, and how will it impact the patient's care? What would you do after researching this question if you were the PA caring for this patient?

• • •

Ben D. Weiss and the Case of Ear Pain

Monday, June 1

2:00 PM

Patient: Ben D. Weiss

Age: 8

Dave and Charlie entered room two to see their next patient, Ben Weiss, for evaluation and treatment of right ear pain. Ben was sitting in one of the chairs against the wall and reading a *Scout Life* magazine. His mother was standing next to him and looking at her phone when they walked in.

Dave greeted Mrs. Weiss and introduced himself and Charlie. "Good afternoon, Mrs. Weiss. I'm Dave Harrington. I'm the PA that runs this clinic. This is Charlie. He's a PA student working with me. Dawn tells us that Ben has some ear pain?"

"That's correct. And, please, call me Lori."

"All right, Lori, let's start by getting a little more information. I'm going to let Charlie ask some questions if you don't mind," Dave replied. He motioned to Charlie to start.

"So when did he first start complaining of ear pain?" Charlie asked.

"He woke up last night with ear pain. I gave him some ibuprofen, which seemed to help some, but he still had pain this morning. Then I noticed that it was pretty swollen in the ear canal and there was some yellowish drainage too. I asked the park ranger ..." She glanced to Dave and said, "We're staying at the Pictured Rocks National Lakeshore." She returned her gaze to Charlie. "He told us about this place and suggested Ben be checked out." To Dave she said, "The ranger spoke very highly of you and the clinic."

"You must have spoken with Kirk. If you see him again, tell him I said thank you for the vote of confidence," Dave said with a smile.

"So the pain started last night, was a little better for a while with ibuprofen, but returned in the morning. And you said the ear canal was swollen and there was discharge?" Charlie asked.

"That's right," Lori replied.

"Has he had a fever or a recent cold?" Charlie asked.

"No. He's been acting fine. We've been up here for a week already, and he's been hiking, biking, and swimming nearly every day. He hasn't slowed down," Lori said.

"Has he been swimming a lot lately? Does he wear earplugs or wear earphones in his ears often?" Charlie asked.

"Oh yeah. Definitely. He is in the water from nearly sunup to sundown. And he's always got those earbuds in his ears when he's not in the water. Come to think of it, he hasn't been wearing them the last few days because he said they hurt his ears."

Swimming and frequent use of devices in the ear (such as earphones, earplugs, or hearing aids) are commonly seen as activities that increase the risk of otitis externa. The risk can be higher with trauma from excessive cleaning or scratching in the canal. The trauma can cause abrasions along the canal and increase access for infectious agents in the body (Agius, Pickles, and Burch 1992).

Dave left his post at the door and approached Ben.

"Hey bud, you mind if I take a look at your ear?" Dave asked.

Ben leaned away from Dave in apprehension. "Just don't touch it. You won't touch it, will you?" he asked.

"Does it hurt if you touch your ear here?" Dave asked, pointing to the tragus on his own ear.

Ben nodded.

"Okay, I won't touch it, but I need to look at it. Is that okay? Just turn your head to the left and tilt your ear up. I'll just look. I promise," Dave said.

Ben did as he was told, and Dave nodded. "Yup. Charlie, come take a look." To Ben he said, "No worries bud, he's not going to touch it either."

Dave pointed out to Charlie that the right ear canal was nearly swollen shut and appeared erythematous. He also pointed out some dried residue at the opening of the canal. He told Lori that Ben likely had otitis externa, or swimmer's ear. He'd need some antibiotics and he'd have to avoid swimming for the rest of his trip. He told Ben he'd have to avoid using his earbuds for his phone or tablet as well. Ben didn't seem too happy with the news, but he was encouraged to hear that with the medication he'd be feeling better soon.

Dave and Charlie sent them on their way to the pharmacy in Munising and discussed the case while they waited for their next patient. They discussed the different treatment options, different causes, and potential preventative measures for swimmer's ear. It wasn't hard for Charlie to come up with some good research questions from the case.

ASSIGNMENT

Come up with a foreground (PICO) question based on this case. Find a study that answers your question, and appraise it for its Validity, Importance, and Usefulness. Use the worksheet in the appendix, and write a brief summary of the study, why you feel it answers your question adequately, and whether the study was valid, important, and useful in this case. What are some of the pros and cons of the study, and how will it impact the patient's care? What would you do after researching this question if you were the PA caring for this patient?

. . .

Marie K. Theoret and the Case of Dysuria

Monday, June 1

2:30 PM

Patient: Marie K. Theoret

Age: 32

Dave and Charlie saw the last patient of the afternoon together. Dave planned to ask the questions and have Charlie do the physical exam. They were seeing Marie Theoret, a 32-year-old woman who was in the office for a urinary tract infection. Dawn had already obtained a urine sample and dipped it before they entered the room, so they knew she had an infection. Her urine dip indicated 2+ leukocytes, positive nitrites, and blood. Dave told Dawn to keep the urine sample so that they could send it to the lab for a culture.

> Urine dips (urinalysis done in the office with a dipstick) are a great way to quickly evaluate for a possible urinary tract infection, but they have some limitations. Be sure your patient has provided a "clean catch, midstream" to prevent contamination. A set of results with blood and leukocytes are common with urinary tract infections but are possible in the absence of true infection. Urine cultures are the preferred test to confirm diagnosis. When nitrites are present, the likelihood of infection by *Enterobacteriaceae* is very high.

When they entered the room, Ms. Theoret was seated in the chair next to the table.

"Good afternoon, Marie," Dave said.

"Hey, Dave. Thanks for getting me in on such short notice. You just opened up the clinic for the season today, right?" she said.

"That's right, and we opened this season with some extra help. This is Charlie. He's a PA student who'll be working here with me for a few months. He's here from downstate," Dave introduced Charlie.

"First time in the U.P.?" she asked.

Charlie nodded. "Yes, ma'am."

"Welcome to the area. I hope you made time for seeing the sights. Summer is beautiful up here."

"Thanks, and I totally plan on seeing everything the U.P. has to offer," Charlie replied with a grin.

Dave sat down at the table. "So, we've already had a look at your urine sample. You've definitely got a urinary tract infection. What kind of symptoms have you had?" Dave asked.

"Well, it hurts to pee for one. I've also got some pain in the back on the right side, and I have to pee all the time. But the funny thing is, when I go to pee, I barely seem to get any to come out. It's super annoying ... and painful," she said.

"Any fever or chills?" Dave asked.

"Nah. I don't think so. But I guess it'd be hard to tell since I take ibuprofen for my feet every night. They really get barking when you've been waitressing on your feet all day."

"I can see your point. Are you aware of how you can get UTIs?" Dave asked.

"Yeah. Gotta wipe front to back and pee after sex. I do that every time, I swear."

"Did you know you can get a UTI by holding your urine and not taking bathroom breaks all day?" Dave asked, pointing to her outfit. She was dressed in clothing that revealed her job at Foggy's.

Marie looked down at her outfit and shrugged. "I was busy all weekend and didn't want to miss out on tips. I'll take more bathroom breaks, I promise," she replied.

Charlie was tasked with doing the physical exam portion of the visit. He listened to her heart and lungs, did an abdominal exam that revealed suprapubic tenderness, and found right-sided costovertebral angle tenderness.

Dave and Charlie stepped out of the room to discuss treatment options, and Dave asked Charlie to pick which antibiotic to prescribe for Marie. Charlie was unsure which one was best. Dave ultimately chose medication for Marie but advised Charlie to research treatment options for UTIs.

ASSIGNMENT

Come up with a foreground (PICO) question based on this case. Find a study that answers your question, and appraise it for its Validity, Importance, and Usefulness. Use the worksheet in the appendix, and write a brief summary of the study, why you feel it answers your question adequately, and whether the study was valid, important, and useful in this case. What are some of the pros and cons of the study, and how will it impact the patient's care? What would you do after researching this question if you were the PA caring for this patient?

• • •

A Night Hike

By closing time, Dave and Charlie had seen several cases that sparked discussions and interests. Most cases that trickled in were for minor issues, which was perfect for a first day on rotation. With easier cases, there was more time to sit and chat. Charlie learned that Dave liked to camp off the trail and hike the trails in the evenings. Charlie mentioned that he was planning to hike down the Pipeline trail after dinner and do some exploring. He was hoping Dave would show him around the local trails.

"I'd love to show you some of the trails, but I can't tonight. I'm heading into Munising to meet someone for dinner. Another night. I promise. Maybe Wednesday? I'll show you where the best blueberries are."

"Sounds good! Any advice on the Pipeline? I'm thinking of taking it into Munising."

"It's pretty straight and level. Gets a little hilly as you get closer to Munising, but it's not too tough of a hike. Shouldn't take too long to get there either. Just watch the weather. I heard it might rain later."

"Thanks for the info!" Charlie packed his stuff into his backpack. "See you tomorrow. Same time?"

"Yup. If you get here by nine o'clock, we can chat on the patio over a coffee. My treat."

"Sounds good! See ya in the morning."

As they left the office, Dave got into his Jeep Wrangler and headed east on M-28 toward Munising. Charlie walked down the road and headed back to his camper.

After having dinner that consisted of beef jerky and toaster pastries from the campground's version of a convenience store, Charlie decided to take his backpack with him on his first evening hike so that he could get some food supplies from Munising at the end of the Pipeline trail. He grabbed his pack, a bottle of water, and his hiking staff before heading out. About the time he was crossing M-28 to enter the Pipeline trailhead, his phone's weather app sounded an alert: a thunderstorm was brewing over Lake Superior and headed his way, bringing fierce winds and rain. Unfortunately, his phone was charging on the counter in his camper, and Charlie had no idea the storm was coming.

* * *

Dave was right. The trail was easy at the start. It was paved for the first 500 yards or so, and then it transitioned to a hard-packed, well-traveled path. There were trail markers every hundred yards or so, but Charlie didn't need to look for them. The trail was easy to recognize, and he found no obvious offshoots into the woods. He had hiked many trails near his home, but had never done any hiking in the U.P. The forest was beautiful. All around the trail stood tall trees with a low underbrush of ferns and fallen leaves beneath. The woods were filled with chirping birds, knocking woodpeckers, and rustling leaves. Charlie didn't understand people who said the woods were quiet. The sounds of the forest seemed to come from every direction.

Early in his hike, the air had been cool. He started the hike wearing jeans, a T-shirt, and a light jacket. But as he ventured further into the woods, the air became muggier, and he found himself shedding the jacket and wishing he had worn shorts. About 40 minutes after he began his hike, he encountered the first signs of change among the surrounding terrain: the path became narrower and started to wind up the side of a hill. After some effort, Charlie found himself near the top of a good-sized hillside overlooking a valley to the south. He could see forest for miles and a small linear clearing off to the west that he thought must be the airfield Dave's Native American friend had mentioned. Behind him and out of his view to the northwest, dark skies threatened on the horizon.

On the other side of the hill, the path began to wind down toward Munising. The distance to the trail's end was only about a quarter mile, and Charlie soon found himself at the end of the trail. The trail ended at the corner of Jasper Avenue and Portage Street. It was there that he realized he had left his phone, with its map features, back at the camper.

From what he remembered, the town was to the right. He took a gamble and headed right, down Jasper Avenue toward town. The dirt road of Jasper Avenue had only a few residential homes along it and soon led Charlie back to M-28 on the outskirts of Munising. Without his phone, he didn't have directions to a grocery store, but after walking this far, turning back empty-handed wasn't an option. He'd simply have to ask for directions when he came to a public establishment. About a half mile down the road, Charlie came across the American Legion. It happened to be across the street from the Tribal Center, and both looked busy tonight. There were several cars parked along the road and the parking lots were full. Charlie headed to the American Legion to request directions. A man smoking a cigarette near the front door nodded to Charlie, who didn't return his recognition at first.

"Out for a hike tonight?" the man asked.

"Mr. Varney! Yes. I'm just checking out the local trails. How's the hand?"

"Better. Beer always helps with pain. You here for a drink?"

"No, just asking directions. I'm looking for a grocery store. You don't happen to know where I can find one, do you?"

"Sorry. I'm new in town too, remember?"

"Right. Well, it was nice seeing you again."

Mr. Varney took another drag on his cigarette and nodded in the direction of the oncoming storm to the northwest.

"You planning on hiking back? Looks like you might get wet."

Charlie followed his gaze and cursed himself for not bringing his phone with the weather app. He nodded and went inside to ask for directions. When he came out, Mr. Varney was gone.

To Charlie's dismay the grocery store was another half mile down the road. This hike had become longer than he anticipated, and now it looked like he would be getting drenched. By the time he exited the grocery store, the sky was noticeably darker and the air was much cooler. Charlie started back to the trail, but as the rain pounded down, he took shelter under the American Legion's awning and was surprised to see Dave exit the bar.

"Charlie! You're all wet. Hiking in the rain?"

Charlie explained his hike to the grocery store, and Dave offered to give him a ride back to the campground. On the way back they chatted about the trail, and Dave agreed to give Charlie a tour of his favorite offshoots of the trail—hiking areas that Charlie must have missed. Charlie asked if Dave had seen Mr. Varney at the American Legion. Dave said he met with a friend for dinner and a drink but didn't see Mr. Varney.

Back at his camper, Charlie found his phone on the counter. He put away his groceries and fired up his laptop to research his PICO questions. The Wi-Fi at the campground was weak, but it worked enough for his needs. He was determined to impress Dave in the morning with the information he found.

CHAPTER 2

Tuesday

A Rainy Morning

On Tuesday, Charlie woke to the sound of rain outside his camper. It had rained all night after the initial storm passed through the area during his hike into town. He was determined to arrive at the clinic early to present what he learned from his research. When he arrived at the clinic, Dave was on the back patio talking to Joseph under umbrellas. Charlie couldn't make out what they were saying because of the rain. He was quickly spotted by Joseph, who abruptly changed the subject and gave Dave a hug. With a nod from Joseph in Charlie's direction, Joseph was gone.

"Good morning, Charlie," Dave said as he approached. "You're here early. I didn't expect to see you till closer to nine o'clock. I didn't get a chance to grab our coffees yet."

"That's all right. I wanted to talk about my research on insulins and burns as we discussed yesterday."

"Sound's great, but it's raining, and Dawn won't be here for another forty-five minutes or so to let us in. What do you say we head over to the coffee shop, have a coffee to warm up, and talk there about what you've learned?"

"Sure!"

They headed into Christmas in a steady rain, which made it hard to see the man waiting on the side of the office building. A pickup truck pulled up and rolled down the driver's side window. The man walked up to the window, handed a brown paper lunch bag through the open window to the driver, and walked across the street to disappear down the Pipeline trail.

. . .

Dave and Charlie returned to the office at 10:20 a.m., a little late for the opening of the office, but they could afford to come late some days with the patient load usually under ten for the day.

Dawn was at the reception desk with her face buried in her phone when they walked through the front door. "You've got a patient in room one and a guest in room two who wants a word with you," she remarked without looking up from her phone.

"A guest?" Dave asked.

Dawn shrugged her shoulders and finally broke her trance from the phone to look at them. "Some guy who says he knows you and you told him recently to show up here if he needs any help." She returned her stare to the phone. "Looks strung out to me."

"All right. Charlie, why don't you go talk to whoever is in room one ..."

"Kid with the runs," Dawn interrupted without looking at them.

"... to the patient with diarrhea, and I'll see about the other guy. Meet me in ten minutes or so to discuss your patient in my office. Sound good?"

"Good by me!" Charlie replied.

With that, Dave took off his coat and went into the room on the right. Charlie took off his raincoat as well, grabbed his gear and a notepad, and entered room one.

● ● ●

Gage W. Herman Has Diarrhea

Tuesday, June 2

10:20 AM

Patient: Gage W. Herman

Age: 13

Room one was the largest patient room in the clinic. It served as the surgical suite and consultation room as well as a patient care room. The room was filled with people, which caught Charlie off guard. He could see why Dawn put them in the largest exam room. Lying on the exam table was a boy who looked to be about thirteen years old. He was in the fetal position and moaning. Four boys of similar age and size lined the wall, all in Boy Scout uniforms. Seated in the patient chair was an older man, maybe in his sixties, who also wore a Boy Scout uniform.

"Hi. My name is Charlie, and I'm a PA student working with Mr. Harrington for the month." Charlie quickly glanced at all the faces in the room and settled on the boy on the table. "This must be Gage." He looked back to the older man and asked, "What prompted you guys to bring him in today?"

Gage answered only with moaning. His Scout leader spoke for him.

"He started having some serious diarrhea last night, followed by a fever, sweats, and shakes. With the quick onset of symptoms, I wanted to be sure he received treatment soon."

"How's he been this morning so far?" Charlie asked.

The tallest boy against the wall spoke up this time. "He hasn't eaten anything today, and he's had some real smelly farts and diarrhea. I mean some real foul stuff. He's been complaining of bad cramps, and he hasn't been able to do much."

"We've been hiking for the past week from Tahquamenon Falls. No one else has been sick so far," the Scout leader added.

"Where have you guys been getting your water?" Charlie asked.

"We get it from hand pumps along the trail when they are available at campsites, but usually we get it from streams and stuff. We add Tang so it don't taste so bad," replied the tall Scout.

"They use water purifying pumps if that's what you're getting at," added the Scout leader.

"Is there any chance Gage didn't use a pump at some point?" Charlie asked.

"That's not likely. I have reiterated a number of times the importance of purifying the water before drinking it."

A young Scout along the wall slowly raised his hand.

"What is it, young man?" Charlie asked.

"Well, when we were at the Falls, Gage and I took a drink right from the Falls. We didn't use any purifier. Am I gonna be sick too?" The young Scout looked worried.

"Not necessarily. Sometimes people don't get symptoms. How long ago was this? When were you guys at the Falls?"

"We were there eight days ago," answered the Scout leader.

> *Giardia* infections can occur when hikers drink inadequately filtered water, often from streams, ponds, or puddles. Person-to-person transmission can also occur when infected patients don't practice adequate hand hygiene in the presence of diarrhea.

"That makes sense. I think Gage has an infection from drinking unpurified water. Let me check him over, and then I'll talk with Mr. Harrington about my findings. He'll come in, probably confirm some things, check him over as well, and then we will tell you what Gage needs to get better."

Charlie approached Gage and asked him if it would be okay to look him over. Gage nodded meekly and rolled to his back. Charlie listened and palpated his abdomen. He found hyperactivity on auscultation and moderate tenderness throughout on palpation.

He stepped out of the room and waited for Dave to return from his visit with his guest and give an opinion on the cause of Gage's discomfort.

• • •

Laura M. Perrin and the Question on Managing Allergies

Tuesday, June 2

11:00 AM

Patient: Laura M. Perrin

Age: 38

Charlie and Dave entered room two together to see their next patient, Laura Perrin, who had come in to discuss treatment options for her allergies. As they entered the room, Laura was sitting in the chair against the wall and looking at her phone. As if on cue, she sneezed when they entered the room.

"Bless you!" Dave said, as he walked into the room with Charlie behind him. "Good morning, Laura. This is Charlie. He's a PA student working with me this summer. What can we do for you today?"

Laura blew her nose into a tissue and tossed it in the garbage. She reached in her purse and pulled out a small bottle of hand sanitizer and started rubbing the solution on her hands.

"Morning, Dave. It's just my allergies again. Seems like every June I get this crap. I've tried to keep it in check with some over-the-counter stuff, but I just can't seem to get on top of it. I need to clear this stuff up. It's not good for business," she said.

"What kind of work do you do?" Charlie asked.

"I'm a brewmaster for a brewery in Munising," she said. "Not being able to smell or taste doesn't bode well for making beer."

"I'd suppose not," Dave replied. "Besides feeling stuffy and losing your ability to smell and taste well, what other symptoms are you having?" he asked.

Laura blew her nose again into a fresh tissue before answering. "Well, my sinuses are full, my eyes are itchy and watery, and my ears are plugged up. I'm miserable, Dave."

"What have you done so far for it? You said you were using over-the-counter meds? What have you tried?" Dave asked.

"I'm taking some loratadine, ten milligrams, I think. And I've been using some fluticasone nasal spray. Both are over-the-counter meds. I've gotten a shot of steroids in the past from my regular doctor. Is that an option?"

"Well, there are some instances where steroid shots have been given to patients for allergies, but there are several other options for allergies that don't involve a shot. Have you tried any other oral medications for allergies in the past—like the brands Zyrtec, Allegra, or Xyzal? Sometimes trying a different medication brand can make your symptoms better. Or have you tried different types of nasal sprays? Have you considered allergy testing or allergy shots? We don't do that here in the clinic, but I could put a referral in for you to have that done if you are interested," Dave said.

Laura shook her head. "I've tried other pills from the pharmacy. None seem to work well for me. I've even tried Benadryl. That works pretty good, but it makes me drowsy. I really just need to clear out my sinuses so I can breathe again and smell. Smelling is super important in my job." She reached in her purse and pulled out a small bottle of Afrin, an over-the-counter nasal decongestant spray. "A friend suggested I try this. She says it works pretty well. I haven't tried it yet because I'm leery about starting anything new that may or may not mess up my smeller. What are your thoughts?"

"Well, nasal sprays like that work well, but can sometimes cause rebound congestion. I'd only use them in emergency situations or very sparingly. Never use them for more than three days in a row," Dave said.

> When prescribing nasal sprays to patients, be sure to instruct them on the proper technique for nasal spray use. When used incorrectly, the nasal spray may be uncomfortable, less effective, and lead to therapy noncompliance. Instead of "snorting" the sprayed medication, instruct the patient to aim the spray nozzle back and away from the nasal septum. Don't tilt the head back because this causes the medication to run down the back of the throat. Lightly sniffle in after each spray. Effectiveness and compliance with taking the medication both improve greatly with proper use.

Laura dropped the bottle in the garbage. "Yeah ... I'm out. Not gonna mess with that. I'll do whatever you suggest, Dave. You know I trust your judgment. You've done me right in the past, so you're all right in my book."

"There are a few treatments we can do for allergies. How about this: let me step out in the hall with Charlie and we'll talk about what we can do for you. We'll break down the options and come back with a good plan for you. Sound good?"

"Dave, you get this to clear up, and I'll give you each a beer on the house the next time you stop in," Laura replied with a smile.

ASSIGNMENT

Come up with a foreground (PICO) question based on this case. Find a study that answers your question, and appraise it for its Validity, Importance, and Usefulness. Use the worksheet in the appendix, and write a brief summary of the study, why you feel it answers your question adequately, and whether the study was valid, important, and useful in this case. What are some of the pros and cons of the study, and how will it impact the patient's care? What would you do after researching this question if you were the PA caring for this patient?

• • •

Ronald G. Wedig and the Case of Alcoholism and Cirrhosis

Tuesday, June 2

11:30 AM

Patient: Ronald G. Wedig

Age: 64

Around 11:30, Dawn poked her head into Dave's office and informed Dave and Charlie that they had a patient waiting in room three. A husband and wife were here to discuss the husband's sudden weight gain.

Dave and Charlie entered the room together and were greeted by Mr. Wedig, a large man with faded tattoos on his arms and an unkempt head of white hair. His beard, white with yellowing from smoking, appeared disheveled as well. He was sitting on the exam table with his arms crossed and looked less than pleased to be here. His wife, Carol, sat in the chair in the corner of the room and stood to greet them when Charlie closed the door behind them.

"Thank you for seeing Ron today, doctor. I'm worried he might be sick." She practically tripped over her own words as she eagerly shook Dave's hand with her two hands clasping his.

"I'm fine, Carol. Just sit down so we can get this charade over with," grunted Ron.

"We're glad to see him, ma'am. I'm Dave Harrington; I'm a PA. This is Charlie. He's a PA student who is working with me for a few months. Please, sit."

After everyone was seated, Dave turned to Mr. Wedig and asked, "What can I do for you today?"

"Why don't you ask her? She made the appointment. There's nothing wrong with me. I'm fine," Ron replied. With his arms still crossed, he turned to glance out the window while looking irritated.

"It's his belly," Carol nearly whispered.

"There's nothing wrong with my stomach! I'm just getting fat!" Ron pinched the bridge of his nose and squeezed his eyes shut in annoyance.

"It's not fat, Ron. You can't get that fat in only two weeks," Carol retorted. Turning her attention back to Dave, she spoke in a hushed voice, "I think it's from his drinking."

Mr. Wedig returned his gaze to the window and the waves of the bay beyond it.

"I see," Dave said. And to Mr. Wedig, "Ron, may I call you Ron?"

Mr. Wedig flipped his right hand dismissively.

"Ron, I've seen you down at the Legion before. Do you go there often?"

"He goes there almost every night," Carol chimed in.

"I'd like Ron to answer my questions for now, Mrs. Wedig, if you don't mind." Returning his attention to Mr. Wedig, "Have you been asked to cut down on your drinking before, Ron?"

"No. It's nobody's business but mine."

"Have you ever felt annoyed by people talking about your drinking or guilty about how much you drink?"

Pointing to Carol he replied, "She annoys me plenty about it. Guilty? Hell no. Drinkin's all I've got now."

Dave asked Mr. Wedig several more questions about his drinking habits and symptoms related to his newly rotund belly. At Dave's encouragement Charlie asked a few questions too, and together they learned that Mr. Wedig was once a Pictured Rocks boat tour captain but was fired a few years back after he was involved in an accident on the water. Apparently, a kayaker was hit by his boat when he wasn't paying attention. Luckily, nobody was seriously injured, but there was a threat of a lawsuit. The suit was dropped when the touring company fired Mr. Wedig. After that he started spending his time at the American Legion, and his drinking steadily became more commonplace. Now he starts each morning with a beer for breakfast and spends each afternoon at one of the several bars in the area. Occasionally, he'll find himself at the Kewadin Casino.

Mr. Wedig's abdomen started to swell slowly at first, likely from the excessive caloric intake of his drinking. Over the past few weeks, however, his abdomen began to swell rapidly, causing his wife to become more concerned. She had been concerned about his drinking for a while, but the sudden change in his appearance caused her alarm. Not only was his abdomen round and appearing ready to explode, his skin had begun to have a yellowish tinge and his breathing had been more labored. He had also recently started complaining of severe leg cramps.

Charlie was asked to start the physical exam. He covered most of the common exam tests, such as listening to the heart and lungs, checking for lymphadenopathy, and examining the mouth. Dave stepped in to do the abdominal exam initially, but let Charlie repeat everything he did. He checked and found a fluid wave and noticed the liver and spleen were both enlarged.

Dave asked if it would be all right if he and Charlie stepped out to discuss their findings and plan for treatment. In the hallway, they discussed ascites, liver disease, alcoholism, and depression. It was clear to both men that Mr. Wedig had all of these conditions. Testing and treatment options were discussed. Ultimately, Mr. Wedig was referred to the gastroenterologist in Marquette. Labs and imaging were ordered so that they would be done before the appointment with the specialist. He was also given a referral to a counselor in Munising to discuss his depression and drinking problem.

Dave thought this case was a prime case for discussing research again. He and Charlie had discussed ascites treatments and found there were differing opinions on whether a combination of spironolactone with furosemide or sequential therapy of the two was the better approach. They also discussed medications used to encourage abstinence of alcohol, like baclofen or Antabuse. They debated depression medications as well. Charlie was charged with researching some of these topics and reporting back the following day with his findings on the evidence.

ASSIGNMENT

Come up with a foreground (PICO) question based on this case. Find a study that answers your question, and appraise it for its Validity, Importance, and Usefulness. Use the worksheet in the appendix, and write a brief summary of the study, why you feel it answers your question adequately, and whether the study was valid, important, and useful in this case. What are some of the pros and cons of the study, and how will it impact the patient's care? What would you do after researching this question if you were the PA caring for this patient?

. . .

Jessica M. McCoy and the Case of Narcotic Bowel Syndrome

Tuesday, June 2

1:40 PM

Patient: Jessica M. McCoy

Age: 22

Dave and Charlie entered room two together to see the first patient of the afternoon. Seated on the exam table was Jessica McCoy, a Munising resident Dave was very familiar with. She had a regular doctor in town, but from time to time, she liked to be treated at Tourist Park Urgent Care Center to keep her private issues private. Despite HIPAA, word tended to get around about patients in a small town like Munising. Tourist Park Urgent Care Center had a reputation of being discrete. She had been taking Norco for neck pain following a kayaking incident where she was hit by a tour boat a few years back. She liked to get her refills from Dave to avoid sideways glances in town.

"Good afternoon, Jessie. This is Charlie. He's going to be working with me for the next couple months. Do you mind if he sits in on the appointment today?" Dave asked.

Jessica looked at Charlie with suspicious eyes and replied, "So long as he doesn't blab to folks around here as to what I'm doing here."

"Nothing leaves this room, ma'am," Charlie said.

"Ma'am? I ain't no old lady! Hell, we're probably the same age." Jessica grimaced and crouched forward, cradling her abdomen.

"You all right, Jessie?" Dave asked.

"No. I think I need my meds increased. I've got stomach pains now on top of my neck pain. I know I'm not supposed to take more than prescribed, but the pain is just too much! I took two Norco this morning, but the stomach just seems to be getting worse. I don't know what to do. I *need* more, Dave!"

"Let me ask you some questions before we talk about your dosage, all right? When did the belly pain start?"

"I get backed up sometimes because of the meds, ya know? So I took some stool softeners like you told me, but it hasn't helped. It seems the pain gets worse despite the increased Norco. It's been like this for a few weeks. I just can't do this anymore. What can I do?"

"Jessie, we just opened the clinic for the season, so where have you been getting your scripts?"

"I gotta be honest, Dave. I get them off the street. I don't take anything else, I promise. I try to take them the same way you wrote them for me, but sometimes the stuff I get is stronger."

"Okay. First, getting them off the street is not safe. Stop buying drugs from a dealer. If you get your Norco from anywhere, it should only be from me or another licensed provider. It's better for everyone if you do that. Second, I think you may have Narcotic Bowel Syndrome."

"What the hell is that, and how do you treat it?"

"There's a way we can make you feel better, but I don't think you're gonna like it," Dave replied.

"I'll do anything. Try me. Just make this pain go away."

Dave explained to Jessica and Charlie that Narcotic Bowel Syndrome was a condition that can be common among patients who use opioid medications regularly. It is a disorder characterized by chronic, recurrent abdominal pain that is worsened by increased frequency or dose of the opioid used to treat it. The only successful treatment is careful weaning off the opioid drug.

Dave and Charlie stepped into the hall to discuss methods for weaning a patient off Norco and alternatives for treating her neck pain, which was the original reason she was prescribed Norco. They talked about medications that may be used to help with the weaning process, including antidepressants and clonidine.

* * *

Alissa D. Hulett and the Question of ADD Management

Tuesday, June 2

2:00 PM

Patient: Alissa D. Hulett

Age: 22

Dave sent Charlie into room three to see Alissa Hulett, who was in the office to get refills of her Adderall for Attention Deficit Disorder (ADD). Alissa, a Northern Michigan University student, started seeing Dave for her Adderall refills when she spent last summer working as an education intern for Pictured Rocks National Lakeshore. She usually had the prescriptions filled on campus in Marquette, but because she spent her summers in Munising, she liked to see Dave. This summer she was back as a paid employee of the National Park Service and again needed refills.

"Good afternoon, my name's Charlie, and I'm a PA student working with Mr. Harrington this summer. I hear you're here today to get refills of some medications?"

"Hey Charlie, I'm Alissa. Nice to meet you. Yeah, I need my Adderall refilled. Should be a pretty straightforward visit," Alissa replied.

"So how long have you been taking Adderall?" Charlie asked.

"I don't know, about four years or so? I was diagnosed when I started at Northern. I really struggled with studying when I got to college, and the doc at the school clinic said I had ADD. She put me on Adderall, and it really helped. I can stay on task and finish projects when I take it. It helps me at school and here at the Park Service. It helped me keep my weight down at school too. It keeps me from wanting to snack all the time."

"Sounds like it might be suppressing your appetite. Do you tend to skip meals because of it? I mean, do you ever forget to eat a meal because of the Adderall?" Charlie asked.

"No. Not really. I mean, sure, I suppose I probably skipped breakfast or only had a cup of coffee in the morning from time to time because I was in a hurry or something, but it's not like I'm only eating one meal per day or anything like that. My campus doc warned me it could make me less hungry. She told me it was important to still eat something, even if it wasn't much. But I'll tell you, it is a good way to keep the weight off while in school. I actually have a tougher time with it in the summer because it's hard to eat a lot when you're working in the woods on the trails all day. I bring snacks with me, but often I forget to eat them when I get so busy." Alissa shrugged. "I guess that's really the only issue I have with my Adderall—not wanting to eat much in the summer months."

"Have you had any other issues with the Adderall? Any problems with your blood pressure? Any headaches, or palpitations?" Charlie asked.

"No, not really."

"How about any dry mouth, constipation, or sleep trouble?"

"Well, I do get dry mouth from time to time, but I drink a lot of water so that usually takes care of it. I only have problems falling to sleep if I take my second dose too late in the afternoon," Alissa replied.

Charlie wrote her responses down, and then asked if she had ever tried other medications for her ADD. She said she hadn't. Charlie told her that he would talk to Dave about her Adderall and her appetite issues. He said there may be another medication that might be a better fit for her—one that doesn't cause loss of appetite. He was thinking of the non-stimulant drug options for ADD. He assumed the stimulant action of the Adderall, which is found in most ADD medications, was to blame for the lack of appetite. He wondered if a non-stimulant medication for ADD would be a better fit.

Charlie thanked Alissa for letting him see her and left to talk to Dave about the case.

When Dave returned from visiting with Alissa, he told Charlie that Alissa had decided not to switch medications because she didn't want to disrupt the benefits of the medication, despite the few side effects. He told Charlie that the idea of switching to a non-stimulant was a reasonable alternative, however.

"In fact, why don't you look up some research on this topic. I'd like to see what you find," Dave told him with a wink.

ASSIGNMENT

Come up with a foreground (PICO) question based on this case. Find a study that answers your question, and appraise it for its Validity, Importance, and Usefulness. Use the worksheet in the appendix, and write a brief summary of the study, why you feel it answers your question adequately, and whether the study was valid, important, and useful in this case. What are some of the pros and cons of the study, and how will it impact the patient's care? What would you do after researching this question if you were the PA caring for this patient?

• • •

Delmont B. McAfee Has Diarrhea Too!

Tuesday, June 2

3:00 PM

Patient: Delmont B. McAfee

Age: 47

Dave and Charlie entered room one to see the last patient of the afternoon, Delmont McAfee, who was in the office to be evaluated for diarrhea.

"Good afternoon, Mr. McAfee. My name is Dave Harrington. I'm a PA here at the clinic, and this is Charlie. He's a PA student working with me today."

"Del. Call me Del."

"All right, Del. I hear you've had some trouble with diarrhea?" Dave asked.

"I've had a little more than just some trouble. I've had the worst case of diarrhea I've ever had," Del replied.

"What makes this diarrhea the worst you've ever had?" asked Charlie.

"It's super watery, smells awful, and I feel horrible. I've got stomach cramps, no appetite, and I think I might have a low-grade fever," Del replied.

"How long have you had the diarrhea?" asked Dave.

"It started three days ago. I had just finished some antibiotics for a sinus infection. I'm glad to get rid of the sinus pain, but this is horrible."

"You just finished some antibiotics for a sinus infection? What did you take?" Dave asked.

"Levofloxacin. It took two rounds of the stuff to knock it out. I called my doc back home in Detroit and he called it in for me. I always seem to get a sinus infection when I get up here. I come up here every summer to go fishing for a few weeks. Usually a course of antibiotics and some nasal spray will kick it, but this year I needed two rounds of antibiotics. I'm all better now with the sinus crud, but this diarrhea is awful."

Dave nodded and put on some gloves. "You mind if I take a look at ya, Del?" Dave asked as he pulled his stethoscope out of his pocket and approached the patient.

"Do whatever it is you need to do to make me better, man," Del replied.

Dave listened to Del's heart and lungs, then had him lie down to listen and palpate his abdomen. His bowel sounds were hyperactive, and the abdomen was moderately tender to palpation.

"Well, I'd say the most likely cause of your diarrhea was actually your antibiotic use. You could have C. Diff," Dave said.

"What's C. Diff?" asked Del.

"It's an infection caused by antibiotics that have disrupted the normal bacteria environment in the colon. Prolonged use of antibiotics like the Levofloxacin can cause it," Charlie said.

"We can treat it with a different antibiotic. Where would you like the script sent?" Dave asked.

. . .

Dave and Charlie discussed the different treatment options after the appointment. They also discussed testing and options for diagnosing C. Diff infections.

> **ASSIGNMENT**
>
> Come up with a foreground (PICO) question based on this case. Find a study that answers your question, and appraise it for its Validity, Importance, and Usefulness. Use the worksheet in the appendix, and write a brief summary of the study, why you feel it answers your question adequately, and whether the study was valid, important, and useful in this case. What are some of the pros and cons of the study, and how will it impact the patient's care? What would you do after researching this question if you were the PA caring for this patient?

. . .

A Stroll on the Beach

The afternoon schedule was pretty light, so Dave, Charlie, and Dawn decided to close the clinic a little early and enjoy the return of good weather. The rain had stopped around noon, and the clouds were now gone, revealing a deep blue sky. It was finally warming up as well. Charlie had gone back to his camper and was doing his research and studying on a nearby picnic table to soak up as much of the warm late afternoon sunlight as possible.

Charlie couldn't stop thinking about what Dave had said about the drug and alcohol problem that was common around Munising. Apparently, drugs and alcohol were becoming more and more a problem everywhere in the U.P., much like everywhere else in the U.S. Dave told Charlie that alcoholism had always been an issue here, with long, cold winters and a struggling economy at times. Drug use, prescription or illicit, had been on the rise as well. The area had seen an increase in meth and heroin use, and there were rumblings of increased hydrocodone and oxycodone use. The local Chippewa tribe had been reporting increased use of prescription opioids as well. Dave told Charlie that he had seen an increase in requests for narcotic pain medications at the clinic during the past few summers, and several patients seemed to be getting them from questionable sources, like the young woman they had seen earlier.

He decided to go for a walk, but not a long hike. He didn't want to get caught too far away from camp after yesterday's fiasco. So instead of heading to the Pipeline trail again, he walked in the direction of the beach.

He walked along the beach in solitude. There were no campers or tourists here today, and the water was far too cold to swim. Lake Superior only warms up to about forty-one degrees in June, so even the most adventurous child would avoid getting wet for too long. He enjoyed the not-so-quiet quiet that walking alone provided. He listened to the waves crashing gently on the shore and the gulls squabbling overhead. He swore that he could see a bald eagle flying over the bay. He had heard somewhere that several bald eagles nested on Grand Island.

He had been walking about a half hour when he found himself not too far from the Grand Island Ferry dock. The dock is just down the road on M-28 on Grand Island Landing Road. The main ferry dock looked quiet at the moment, but some movement at a nearby shed caught Charlie's attention. He noticed a large man leaning against the shed with his back to Charlie. Then, not long after Charlie spotted the man, an older model gray Chevy Silverado pulled up next to the shed, blocking Charlie's view of the man. When the door opened, Charlie was surprised to see Dawn get out of the truck. She was carrying a large envelope, and she went around the vehicle to meet the man. Charlie's view was obstructed so that he couldn't see what was happening. After only a minute or two, Dawn returned to the truck and drove off. And the man was gone. Charlie thought perhaps he went to the ferry dock, which was starting to get busy as the ferry had come in while the events near the shed unfolded. There were several large men working on the dock, and the man by the shed could easily have slipped among them. *What was Dawn doing out here?* he thought.

Charlie checked his watch. It was past seven. No wonder he was hungry; he hadn't eaten yet. He decided he had better get back to the camper and make dinner. He had more reading to do.

CHAPTER 3

Wednesday

Someone Is Missing in Action

When Charlie arrived at the clinic Wednesday morning, he noticed a minivan parked in front. He had expected to find the truck he saw last night at the dock. He was certain the woman he saw was Dawn, but he had never really paid attention to what vehicle she drove. He thought he remembered seeing her pull up in a silver truck on his first day, but he couldn't be sure. Perhaps his mind was messing with his memory of that morning to make it match what he thought he had seen the previous night. Dave wasn't at the clinic yet, which surprised Charlie. So far, from what he had experienced and been told, Dave liked getting to the clinic early. Seeing an unfamiliar minivan and beating Dave to the clinic gave Charlie an uneasy feeling.

When he entered the office, an older woman looked up from behind the reception desk and raised her eyebrows.

"We open at 10 a.m., dear. You can have a seat if you don't mind waiting."

"Um. I'm Charlie. I'm a PA student working with Dave Harrington," Charlie awkwardly replied.

"Oh. Sorry, dear. You can come on back. Mr. Harrington will be here shortly. He had something to attend to on the way in. My name is Carol Swienhart. I'm a travel nurse filling in for Dawn today. I'm sorry to say she's under the weather. Should be back tomorrow, though. Why don't you have a seat in Mr. Harrington's office and wait for him there? He shouldn't be much longer."

Ms. Swienhart returned her attention to the stack of paperwork in front of her, and Charlie walked back to the office. He put his white coat and bag down on a chair and decided to step out onto the back patio to wait for Dave.

As Ms. Swienhart indicated, Dave arrived a few minutes later. He greeted Charlie as he opened the patio door.

"Good morning, Charlie. Sorry for not being here when you got in. Dawn called in sick, and she rarely ever does, so I decided to check in on her on my way in."

"And? She all right?" Charlie asked.

"Yeah. She's fine. Not even sick. She had a personal family issue come up and needed to head over to Marquette this morning. I got to her place just as she was backing out of her drive. She said she'd be gone all day but should be back to work tomorrow."

Charlie nodded, thinking of what he had seen the previous night and wondering whether her trip to Marquette was related, if the woman indeed was Dawn.

Dave must have interpreted Charlie's look of thoughtfulness as worry about Ms. Swienhart because he said, "Don't worry. Carol is great. I've worked with her before."

"Well, she seems nice," Charlie replied.

Dave and Charlie went into the office to discuss questions and research findings from Tuesday. They discussed treatment options for cirrhosis, ascites, GI tract infections, and opioid management. They talked about drug and alcohol addiction, local hangouts, and hiking. Charlie didn't talk about his hike to the docks, however. He decided to keep what he saw there close to his vest for now.

Shortly after the clinic opened at 10 a.m., Carol popped her head into Dave's office to let them know that the first patient of the morning was here—another Boy Scout, this time with an orthopedic complaint.

. . .

Robert J. Clearwood and the Case of Heel Pain

Wednesday, June 3

10:10 AM

Patient: Robert J. Clearwood

Age: 12

Dave and Charlie entered room one together to see Robert. Dave had decided to let Charlie do all the talking and perform the physical exam while he observed. When he had students see patients in this manner, he usually would only interject and ask more questions if he felt they were needed, but he always repeated the physical exam. Charlie and Dave were greeted by the same group of Boy Scouts and the Scout leader they had seen the day before. Gage, looking a little better today (at least he was not moaning on the table in the fetal position) stood against the wall with three other boys. The Scout leader was again seated in the chair, and a different boy sat on the exam table. Dave stood back against the door and crossed his arms over his chest, ready to listen. Charlie took the seat across from the Scout leader.

"Good morning, everyone. Welcome back to the clinic. I'm Charlie, the PA student. We met yesterday. I'm sure you remember Dave Harrington. He's the PA here at the clinic." Charlie motioned to Dave, who looked to each boy. "Welcome back. What brings you back so soon?"

"I think Robbie here's got plantar fasciitis," replied the Scout leader. "We would have had him seen yesterday, but he's kind of a quiet one. He didn't complain till this morning, after we had a long break on our early morning hike. The boys tell me he's been complaining about his right foot since breakfast. After our hike this morning was the first I heard of it, though."

Turning to the boy on the table, Charlie asked if he'd prefer to be called Robbie.

"All my friends call me that," he answered. He was looking down at his feet and avoiding eye contact.

"May I call you Robbie?"

"Sure."

"Okay. Why don't we start with you telling me where your foot hurts?"

Without looking up, Robbie said, "It don't hurt now. It doesn't hurt all the time."

"Did you injure the foot? Maybe you rolled it or twisted it somehow? Or did you step on something or drop something on it?"

"No. Nothing like that. It hurts on the bottom." He put his right foot up on his left knee and pointed to the bottom of the right heel. "But it only hurt when I got up this morning and after we had a rest when we were on our hike."

"I see," Charlie replied. He placed his thumb over the place where the plantar fascia attaches to the calcaneal tuberosity and gently pressed. "Does this hurt?"

Robbie pulled his foot away and said, "Yes! That's where it hurt when I got out of the tent this morning."

Charlie turned to the Scout leader and confirmed his suspicions. "Yes, I do believe he has plantar fasciitis." To Robbie, he said, "But don't worry, it's treatable, and we'll get you feeling better soon."

The tall Scout who had spoken up the day before said, "See, Robbie? It has nothing to do with any curse."

"What curse would that be?" asked Dave, who was examining Robbie's foot now.

The tall Scout snickered. Another boy answered for him. "We were having a campfire last night and telling ghost stories. Ben told a story about a Scout who was cursed after disturbing an Indian burial site. The Scout in the story had walked over sacred ground and disturbed the offerings. The story told how the Scout slowly lost the ability to walk and move and eventually became a tree in the woods."

"Yeah, and it started in the feet!" added the smallest Scout on the wall.

Dave asked Robbie, "Why would you think your heel pain was part of the curse in the story?"

Robbie looked to the floor, shrugged his shoulders, and said nothing.

"Yesterday afternoon we were hiking a trail between the Pipeline trail and the Old Golf Course Road trail when we saw something that looked a little spooky," replied the tall Scout, who evidently was named Ben.

"I walked right through it and accidentally knocked over a stack of rocks," Robbie added.

"What was so spooky about a stack of rocks?" Charlie asked.

"The boys came across what appeared to be an abandoned campsite. There were ropes hung up with tin cans attached to them that were similar to wind chimes, and three stacks of rocks were spaced about the site. It looked like there was a firepit that hadn't been used in a while and several deer antlers that were cut in pieces lay on the ground by the firepit. It wasn't a graveyard," the Scout leader replied. And to the boys, he said, "And the antlers were *not* offerings. Now why did you have to go and scare Robbie like that?" He shook his head, but couldn't completely conceal his amusement.

Dave looked to Robbie and assured him, "Not a curse, Robbie, just some plantar fasciitis."

Dave advised Robbie to roll a water bottle along the bottom of his foot several times per day to stretch out the plantar fascia. A frozen one would be best if they could get their hands on one. Tennis balls worked well too, but he didn't think the boys would have one in their backpacks. He discussed other stretches that could work and the pros and cons of heel cups versus arch support insoles. He said that the pharmacy in town would have some, but he would see whether he could find some in the sample closet in the office. He also discussed medication options versus injections.

ASSIGNMENT

Come up with a foreground (PICO) question based on this case. Find a study that answers your question, and appraise it for its Validity, Importance, and Usefulness. Use the worksheet in the appendix, and write a brief summary of the study, why you feel it answers your question adequately, and whether the study was valid, important, and useful in this case. What are some of the pros and cons of the study, and how will it impact the patient's care? What would you do after researching this question if you were the PA caring for this patient?

• • •

Carly G. Hightower and the Question on Ankle Injuries

Wednesday, June 3

11:00 AM

Patient: Carly G. Hightower

Age: 24

For their next patient, Charlie was sent in alone to get a history from Carly Hightower, a young female mountain biker that came in with her boyfriend to have her ankle examined. According to Ms. Swienhart, Carly had injured her ankle while biking, and her boyfriend had done his best to stabilize her ankle before bringing her in to have it looked at.

When Charlie entered the room, he saw a young woman sitting on the exam table with two thick branches tied to her lower left leg in an attempt to splint the ankle. Her face was a little pale and streaked with dirty tear tracks. Her breaths shuddered as she inhaled. He thought she must have just finished crying. Her boyfriend stood beside her and held her hand with his left hand while he slowly rubbed her back with his right.

"Good morning, my name is Charlie. I'm a PA student working with Mr. Harrington. He asked me to come in and get some information before he joins us. Do you mind if I ask you a few questions?" Charlie asked.

"Sure," Carly replied, barely keeping her tears from returning.

Charlie set down his clipboard and walked over to the exam table to get a better look at the boyfriend's handiwork. "This looks like a pretty good splint. How'd we end up needing it?" he asked.

"We were riding on some bike trails when she had a spill. I didn't see it, but she said she couldn't put weight on her left ankle, so I found some thick branches and made a splint with straps off our bikes," the boyfriend replied.

"Well, it looks pretty good. The ankle, on the other hand, not so much," Charlie said. He was looking at the amount of discoloration and swelling around the lateral aspect of the ankle. "Do you remember how you injured it?"

"I lost my balance going around a bend, and I remember putting my foot out to brace my fall. I ended up rolling the ankle and crashing anyway," Carly said, wincing at the mention of rolling the ankle. "I swear it felt like it snapped like a twig." Her voice wavered as if she were about to cry before getting herself under control again.

"Did the ankle roll inward, like this?" Charlie asked, demonstrating an inversion of the ankle.

"Yeah, just like that."

"She's lucky the ankle is the only thing she messed up. Somehow, she managed to avoid a few trees and only come up with scratches and a bum ankle," her boyfriend said. "Had to leave the bikes there, though. She couldn't pedal. She said it hurt too bad. So I locked them up to a tree off the trail, and we hobbled back to the car and came right here. You guys have an x-ray machine, right?"

"Actually, no, I don't think we do. But let's not jump the gun yet. Dave has to evaluate her before we think about imaging. Can you tell me where the pain is the worst? Try pointing to the spot that is most painful."

Carly pointed to a spot just above the lateral malleolus. It was very swollen and bruised.

"Do you have pain anywhere else on the foot or the other side of the ankle?" Charlie asked.

"Well, the whole thing hurts, but the pain is definitely worse on this side. I can touch the rest of the foot and ankle and it doesn't kill me, but that spot there is a no-touch zone," she replied, pointing again to the lateral malleolus.

"What have you guys done for the pain so far? Have you taken any over-the-counter pain medications, or applied ice or anything yet?" Charlie asked.

"I took some ibuprofen in the car before we got here," Carly said.

"How many did you take?" Charlie asked.

"I think I took three? Could have been four. I know four is the max, right?"

"Yeah, 800 mg, or four over-the-counter ibuprofen would be the maximum dose. Have you put any ice on the ankle?" Charlie asked.

"No, not yet," the boyfriend replied.

"Alright, well, I'm going to step out now to talk to Dave about your situation, and we'll come back with a plan on whether or not we will need an x-ray today. There are clinical practice guidelines that help us make decisions on whether or not an x-ray is needed in situations like this. I have my suspicions, but I'd rather wait to see what Dave thinks before we decide on the next step.

> Clinical Practice Guidelines are guidelines for practitioners and patients intended to aid in the decisions on appropriate health care practices. They are developed using evidence from multiple sources that have undergone diligent review. The evidence is collected and presented in a way to give the reader a concise, evidence-based suggestion, meant to ease the practitioner's or patient's decisions. Can you find any Clinical Practice Guidelines for ankle injuries?

"I'll bring back some ice for the swelling. If you need anything in the meantime, just poke your head out the door and call for Ms. Swienhart. She can get you whatever you need. I'll be right back."

Charlie stepped out and discussed the case with Dave. They discussed the likelihood of a fracture and Clinical Practice Guidelines to help with determining whether an x-ray would be needed. They also talked about treatment options and predicted outcomes for ankle injuries.

When they returned to the room, they broke the news to Carly and her boyfriend: she'd have to head to Marquette for an x-ray.

ASSIGNMENT

Come up with a foreground (PICO) question based on this case. Find a study that answers your question, and appraise it for its Validity, Importance, and Usefulness. Use the worksheet in the appendix, and write a brief summary of the study, why you feel it answers your question adequately, and whether the study was valid, important, and useful in this case. What are some of the pros and cons of the study, and how will it impact the patient's care? What would you do after researching this question if you were the PA caring for this patient?

* * *

Later that morning, Charlie and Dave entered room two to see a familiar patient, Jason Varney, who was here for a wound debridement of the burn on his left hand.

"Good morning, Mr. Varney. How's the hand?" Dave asked.

"Morning, Sir. The hand is doin' well, but my back hurts something fierce," he replied.

"Let's start with looking at your burn, shall we?" Dave said, ignoring the back comment.

> **Jason K. Varney Returns for a Recheck and Has a Request**
>
> **Wednesday, June 3**
>
> **11:30 AM**
>
> **Patient: Jason K. Varney**
>
> **Age: 37**

Dave waved Charlie over to remove the dressings and do the debridement. To everyone's surprise, the wound was healing faster than expected. Charlie cut away the dead skin, applied more silver sulfadiazine and gauze, and rewrapped the hand.

"Does your hand hurt much?" Charlie asked.

"Not really, kid, but like I said, my back hurts something fierce."

"All right, we can talk about the back now. What's going on? On a scale from zero to ten, what's your pain level?" Dave asked.

"I'd say a twelve, man," he replied, while lounging back in his chair. "Any chance you got something for the pain that's better than naproxen? It'd help me out. I got a long hike ahead of me with a heavy pack."

"Where does it hurt?" asked Charlie.

"Low back, just above the hip on the right. I've got an old injury, compliments of an IED that took out the Humvee I was in back in Afghanistan. I always have a little discomfort, but I did some heavy lifting yesterday morning that tweaked my back."

"What were you lifting? How heavy do you think?" asked Dave.

"I was moving some rocks. They were probably twenty pounds each? I'm not sure."

Dave looked puzzled and asked, "How'd you manage to lift the rocks with only one good hand?"

"Very carefully," Jason replied with a smirk.

Dave proceeded to do a physical exam on Jason, starting with the heart and lungs and eventually covering musculoskeletal and reflexes. Charlie watched and took notes. Dave did a straight leg raise test that was negative, and Jason didn't really exhibit any discomfort until Dave asked the pain scale again "to get it charted." This time the number was an eight.

"Well, based on your exam, I think your naproxen is the best bet for treatment. I could give you some back stretches and exercises if you'd like, and maybe a muscle relaxer," Dave suggested.

"Come on, man. I have it on good authority that I can get Norco from you. It's what I need. Just get me a small script, and I'll be on my way."

Dave stood up and opened the door to the exam room. "You can be on your way because I'm not giving you Norco. Just take the naproxen you have and do stretching. If you're still around by Friday, I'd like to see your hand again. And stop lifting heavy stuff with that hand."

Jason stood up and looked Dave in the eyes. He didn't look angry; rather he looked a little confused, like he expected a different outcome. "All right, man. All right." He headed out the door and looked back to Dave and then to Charlie. He nodded and left.

ASSIGNMENT

Come up with a foreground (PICO) question based on this case. Find a study that answers your question, and appraise it for its Validity, Importance, and Usefulness. Use the worksheet in the appendix, and write a brief summary of the study, why you feel it answers your question adequately, and whether the study was valid, important, and useful in this case. What are some of the pros and cons of the study, and how will it impact the patient's care? What would you do after researching this question if you were the PA caring for this patient?

• • •

Leanne M. Forman, Is This Fibromyalgia?

Wednesday, June 3

1:30 PM

Patient: Leanne M. Forman

Age: 66

Dave and Charlie went together to see their first patient after lunch. They were seeing Leanne Forman, a sixty-six-year-old woman who was in the office seeking relief from her fibromyalgia. She was a new patient to the clinic and was being seen here for the first time. When they entered the room, Ms. Forman was seated in the chair next to the counter with her arms crossed over her chest.

"Good afternoon, Ms. Forman. My name is Dave Harrington. I'm a PA here at the clinic, and this is Charlie, a PA student working with me today. Ms. Swienhart tells me you've been having some pain that just won't go away. Is that right?"

"Yeah, I have fibromyalgia. Do you know what that is?" Without giving Dave a chance to reply, Leanne continued. "I'll tell you what it is, in case you don't know. It's pain all over. I hurt everywhere, all the time. Nothing makes it go away. But my regular doctor from downstate has me on some medicine that seems to help some. It's the only way I can get anything done. I'm here today because I need you to prescribe me the same stuff. I'm here for the next few months, and my doctor says he can't prescribe it to me while I'm up here. He said that because it's a controlled substance I should find someone local to write it."

"Okay, but before we talk about treatments, I'd like to learn a bit more about you and your fibromyalgia. Can you tell me where you hurt the most?" Dave asked.

"Like I said, I hurt everywhere," she replied with an eye roll. "But if I had to say it were worse anywhere in particular, I'd say my arms and shoulders are the worst. My back and legs ache all the time too, but not as bad as my arms and shoulders. I'm sure you've never had pain like this. I've tried everything, and nothing really works but the stuff my doctor gives me, so I don't see why we need to discuss this."

"You said you've had this for a while now. How long is a while?" Dave asked.

Leanne sighed. "I don't know, fifteen, twenty years or so? It's been a long time. I know it's not going to get better. I'm tired all the time, my joints are stiff, and I barely get any sleep anymore. The only thing that helps is Norco."

And there it is, thought Charlie.

"Well, your history certainly suggests fibromyalgia. I'll give you that. I would have to do an exam before we discuss therapy."

"If that's what you have to do so I can get my medication, go right ahead. Seems like a waste of time if you ask me. I know what I have, and I know what works," Leanne replied.

Dave listened to her heart and lungs and did a musculoskeletal exam. Leanne routinely winced and pulled away when he palpated her arms, shoulders, and back, often after light or moderate palpation. Her neurological exam was normal.

With the examination done, Dave discussed different treatment options for fibromyalgia, including exercise programs, tricyclic antidepressants, SNRIs, anti-convulsants, or neuropathic pain medications. She seemed less than impressed. Dave also discussed narcotic use for management of fibromyalgia.

Leanne left the office a little upset that he wouldn't prescribe her narcotics.

"This was not how I saw this visit going," she said. "I need that medication, and from what I've heard around town, this was the place to get it!"

She stormed out of the office while Dave looked on with a look of bewilderment. "What is that supposed to mean?" he asked no one in particular.

Dave and Charlie discussed fibromyalgia management while they waited for their next patient. Charlie decided he'd look closer into it when time allowed.

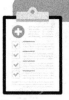

Come up with a foreground (PICO) question based on this case. Find a study that answers your question, and appraise it for its Validity, Importance, and Usefulness. Use the worksheet in the appendix, and write a brief summary of the study, why you feel it answers your question adequately, and whether the study was valid, important, and useful in this case. What are some of the pros and cons of the study, and how will it impact the patient's care? What would you do after researching this question if you were the PA caring for this patient?

⚫ ⚫ ⚫

Bob J. Wright and the Question of Evaluating Sore Throats

Wednesday, June 3

2:30 PM

Patient: Bob J. Wright

Age: 36

For their next patient, Charlie once again accompanied Dave and stood back to observe. They were seeing Bob Wright, a thirty-six-year-old cook from the casino. He was in the office with complaints of a sore throat for the last several days, and he needed a note excusing his work absences.

"Hey, Bob, what brings you in today?" Dave asked as he shook Bob's hand.

"Just need a note for work, man. I missed a few days because of a sore throat. But all's good now," he replied.

"Have a seat, Bob. Let's talk about it," Dave said as he sat in the chair across from Bob's. "So, tell me about this sore throat. Did you have a fever with it?"

Often, a provider will start developing his or her differential diagnosis for a visit prior to heading in to see the patient. The differential diagnosis starts with the chief complaint and can change after more information is ascertained. In this case, Dave and Charlie likely were thinking of an infectious etiology, such as viral illness or streptococcal sore throat. Other diagnosis possibilities, such as irritation from reflux or vomiting, were likely lower. Outside factors, such as recent patient trends, prior history with the patient, or diagnosis frequency often play a role in determining what is at the top of the differential list prior to seeing the patient. As more information is obtained during the visit, the differential diagnosis list changes, and in this case, infectious causes move down the list while others, namely reflux, move up the list.

"Nah, nothing like that. It was pretty bad, though. For like three days in a row, I woke up with a real bad sore throat. It hurt to swallow. Never had a fever, though."

"Any other symptoms, like a cough or headache?" Dave asked.

"Nah, no cough or headache or anything. Well ... I had a hangover the first day, though," he said with a smirk. "We were out partying the night before, and the morning after, I had a bad sore throat and a killer hangover. I guess I just thought it was from all the partying. You know what I'm talking about, right?" he said, holding his hand out for a high five.

Dave left him hanging and shook his head. "So did you drink or party the other nights too? I mean, the nights before your sore throats?"

"Nah, we just partied that first night. I'm too old to party like that every night, man. I just stayed in and watched movies and ate pizza both nights."

"Have you taken any medications to help with your symptoms?" Charlie asked from his position by the door.

Bob looked to Charlie, then back to Dave. "I took some ibuprofen, but it made my stomach hurt so I only took it once."

"Well, I think I know what caused your sore throat," Dave said. "But first, let's have Charlie take a look in your throat and do an exam, okay?"

Charlie looked at his throat, checked his lymph nodes, looked in his ears, and listened to his heart and lungs. Dave repeated the exam and said, "Yup, seems about right. You mind lying on the table so I can check out your abdomen?"

The abdominal exam elicited mild discomfort on moderate to deep palpation of the epigastric region, but was otherwise unremarkable.

"Well, Bob, I think your sore throat was from some GERD," Dave said.

"GERD?" Bob asked.

"Gastroesophageal reflux disease. Some people call it heartburn. I think all the increased acid from your night of drinking and subsequent late nights with pizza caused you to have a sore throat while you lie on your back sleeping. There are some treatment options out there, but for now, I'd like you to avoid tomato-based food, heavy consumption of alcohol, and medications that are irritable to the stomach, like ibuprofen," Dave said.

"You could elevate the head of your bed as well to keep the acid from creeping up while you sleep," Charlie chimed in.

"He's right. You could try that too. In the meantime, I'll send a prescription to the pharmacy for you," Dave said.

Bob said he still needed a note for the days he missed, so Dave jotted down a note excusing his absences.

In the hall after Bob left, Charlie asked Dave which medication class he preferred for treatment of GERD—H2 blockers or proton-pump inhibitors. They discussed the pros and cons of each, and Dave suggested Charlie research it so they could discuss it later.

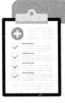

ASSIGNMENT

Come up with a foreground (PICO) question based on this case. Find a study that answers your question, and appraise it for its Validity, Importance, and Usefulness. Use the worksheet in the appendix, and write a brief summary of the study, why you feel it answers your question adequately, and whether the study was valid, important, and useful in this case. What are some of the pros and cons of the study, and how will it impact the patient's care? What would you do after researching this question if you were the PA caring for this patient?

• • •

Mary S. King and Her Wrist Injury

Wednesday, June 3

3:00 PM

Patient: Mary S. King

Age: 62

After having Charlie watch for the first few visits in the early afternoon, Dave decided Charlie needed to see a patient on his own again, so he sent him in to see Mrs. Mary King. Mrs. King was a long-time friend of Dave's who worked at the American Legion. She was on the schedule to be seen for arthritis and severe pain in her left wrist after a recent fall.

"Good afternoon, Mrs. King. My name is Charlie; I'm a PA student working with Mr. Harrington this summer. Thanks for letting me talk to you today."

"It's nice meet you, Charlie. I'm always willing to see Dave's students. You've got to learn somewhere, and with all my health issues, you certainly can learn a thing or two from seeing me."

"So what brings you into the clinic today?" asked Charlie.

"Well, I had a little fall the other day, and I hurt my wrist in the process. It's been more than a week, and the pain isn't going away. I'm afraid I might have broken something. I'm used to pain. I've got the 'arther' just about everywhere. I take meloxicam every day for that, but it doesn't seem to do a thing for my wrist," she said, raising her left wrist to indicate her injured limb. It was wrapped in an elastic bandage. "Dave's told me before that I shouldn't take any other NSAIDs while on my medicine, so I took some acetaminophen for the pain. I have for days, but it hasn't helped at all."

"When did you fall?" Charlie asked.

"A week ago yesterday. I was cleaning up at the Legion after we closed early. There was a fight in the bar that night." She shook her head. "It was all over some girl, and it was getting late. Things can get out of hand when it gets late at the bar," she sighed. "Anyway, I was cleaning up and slipped on some spilled beer. I fell back and tried to catch myself with my left arm. I had my arm out straight with the hand on the floor, like this." She demonstrated an outstretched arm with a flat palm to the floor. "I thought I sprained it at first, but now I'm not so sure."

"Where does it hurt?"

"Here," she said, rubbing the palmar side of the hand at the base of the thumb, over the scaphoid bone.

"Well, let's have a look at it." Charlie gently took Mary's hand and went through some range-of-motion testing and palpated the hand and wrist. He did a test for snuffbox tenderness that was positive. He nodded knowingly. "Looks like you might have a scaphoid fracture, Mrs. King."

> Whenever you have a patient fall on an outstretched arm, you should consider a scaphoid fracture. That is the most common carpal bone fracture and usually occurs after a fall. The pain is usually reported on the radial aspect of the wrist at the base of the thumb. Because of relatively high risk for neuromuscular compromise with open fractures of the scaphoid bone, early recognition, imaging, and surgical intervention should be considered (Alshryda et al. 2012).

"What do we do about that?" she asked.

"Well, I'll have to have Dave take a look and see what he thinks, but we probably will get an x-ray, and you'll probably need to see a hand specialist or an orthopedist. We'll have to cast it or put you in a splint likely. I'm not sure what he'll do for the pain. Norco, maybe?"

"Well, I don't want any of that Norco garbage. I've seen too many good kids around here fall prey to that junk. That's what that girl the boys were fighting over died from—an overdose on Norco or something like that. That grieving boy should never had picked a fight with that big fella. I'm sure you guys saw the boy in here after. Dave said he fixed him up."

"I don't know. I just started here on Monday. I wasn't here last week," Charlie replied.

"Well, Dave's been taking that boy under his wing ever since. I've seen him talking to him a few times at the Legion."

Charlie nodded and thought about each time Dave said he was meeting someone, as well as a guest visiting him in the clinic yesterday. He thought the injured guy might be the person Dave was meeting with.

Charlie stood and headed to the door. Turning back to address Mrs. King, he said, "Well, let me get Dave in here to take a look and see if he agrees with my plan for your wrist. I'll be back soon."

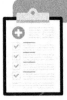

Come up with a foreground (PICO) question based on this case. Find a study that answers your question, and appraise it for its Validity, Importance, and Usefulness. Use the worksheet in the appendix, and write a brief summary of the study, why you feel it answers your question adequately, and whether the study was valid, important, and useful in this case. What are some of the pros and cons of the study, and how will it impact the patient's care? What would you do after researching this question if you were the PA caring for this patient?

• • •

Finally Exploring Some Trails

After work that evening Charlie was exhausted. The day had been a busy one in the clinic. He was glad the clinic closed at 6 p.m., leaving him plenty of quality daylight to enjoy the nature that was all around and still get his studying finished. He was hoping to hike down the trails and see if he could find the "spooky" campsite the Scouts had mentioned. While Charlie was packing up his bag, Dave came into the office and asked what his plans were for the evening.

"Studying, of course," Charlie replied with a grin. "And maybe a little hiking on the trails. It's too nice not to head out there. I've only been on the Pipeline so far. I was thinking of shooting over to the Old Golf Course Road trail."

"Mind if I join you?" Dave asked. "I could show you some of the offshoots on the trail where Joe and I have done some trail restoration. Maybe see if we can find this mysterious Indian burial ground?" he said with a smirk.

"You think we could find it?" Charlie replied.

"Yeah. It sure sounds like an abandoned campsite. Funny thing is, I've been out there nearly every day for weeks, until this week anyway, but I've never seen anything like what they were describing. I'd like to check it out."

"I'd love it if you showed me around the trails. Let's meet up at the Pipeline trailhead in an hour or so? I'll need to change and get a bite to eat first," Charlie said.

• • •

Dave was already at the trailhead when Charlie arrived shortly after seven. Apparently, he had changed at the clinic. He said he kept a change of clothes at the clinic for those nights when he wanted to hike on the trails. They walked about a mile down the trail before Dave found the path to a ravine on the right side of the trail that led to a trail out of view from the Pipeline. It was easy to miss if you didn't know what to look for. Today it looked more obvious, thanks to the earlier trampling of the leaves and grass by the Scouts.

They hiked for about an hour along the trail until they came across a stream. After the heavy rains on Monday night and Tuesday, the stream was flowing at a good pace. The trail had no bridge or crossway, and it looked like hikers usually just hopped across a few strategically placed rocks. With the higher water level, that looked to be a bit difficult.

"We'll have to find a better place to cross. You head downstream to see if there's a better place, and I'll go upstream. Yell if you find a better place, but don't go too far. If there isn't a good way to cross, we'll just abandon the idea," Dave said.

Charlie walked about 200 yards downstream. It didn't seem to look any easier to cross downstream. It actually looked worse. There was a downed tree partway across the stream, but it wouldn't hold their weight, and even if it did, it would only take them about halfway across.

Giving up hope, Charlie started back to the trail. That's when he heard Dave yell out that he had found something. When Charlie caught up with Dave, he was standing at the edge of a clearing on the water's edge about 300 yards upstream.

"This must be the site the Scouts were talking about. They must have found it while looking for a way to cross," Dave said.

They were standing on the edge of a clearing that was about twenty feet in diameter. Three stacks of rocks, each three or four feet tall, were spread out around the site. They created a formation that reminded Charlie of Stonehenge, but in a triangle pattern instead of a circle. One of the piles had been knocked over. Surrounding the circular clearing were dozens of beer cans on fishing lines dangling from trees. They hung in various lengths, with some reaching the ground and others at chest or head height. There was a firepit in the middle with a flattened area next to it, probably from a tent. Next to the firepit was a pile of small sticks and logs, as well as half a dozen deer antlers, some chopped but most intact. Flecks of metal shavings were also near the firepit.

"Looks like a campsite. You think the cans are a form of "security" measure to know if someone comes in the site?" Charlie asked.

"Probably," Dave replied. He looked disappointed. "I've seen this type of campsite before."

"Oh yeah? Where?"

"It's not important, but let's get out of here before the person staying here returns," Dave said, turning to head back to the main trail.

Dave said nothing about the site on the hike back and changed the subject whenever Charlie hinted of bringing it into conversation. Instead, they talked about trail conservation, Charlie's rotation, musculoskeletal issues, the local opioid issues, and music.

When they returned to the trailhead, it was getting dark. Charlie would only have a few hours to research his PICO questions from the day. Dave returned to the clinic to get his Jeep and go home, while Charlie went back to his camper. He'd been here for only three days, and already he had a lot of questions, both clinical and about the happenings in the quiet U.P.

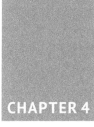

CHAPTER 4

Thursday

Returning to the Scene

Charlie was up, dressed, and already on the Pipeline trail by 7 a.m. Thursday morning. After finding answers to his Wednesday PICO questions, Charlie often found his thoughts drifting back to the abandoned campsite they had found. He had so many questions that needed answering. So he had decided the night before that he was going to get up early and head back out to the site to get another look before the clinic opened at 10 a.m. He ate a breakfast consisting of granola bars and water while he searched for the trail leading to the site. The day before it had only taken close to a half hour to get back from the site, so he figured he would have plenty of time to snoop around. To his dismay, it took him nearly a half hour to find the trail that broke off the Pipeline. He hadn't planned on it taking so long to find the trail. When he reached the stream, it was already 8:30 a.m. That only left about a half hour for snooping. He still wanted to reserve enough time to get back to the clinic before it opened.

The site looked to Charlie to be unchanged from the day before. The stones hadn't been moved, the cans still hung from fishing line, and the firepit looked unused. He looked at the firepit a bit more closely and noted metal shavings among the ashen logs. He picked up an antler and noticed it was hollowed out and had been cut to be about three inches in length. He walked around the site looking to the ground for any bits of garbage or clues as to who might have been here. He found a few items among the leaves: cigarette butts, some pieces of twine, a neckerchief slide (*probably a Scout's*, Charlie thought), and a partial matchbook with the name Kewadin Casinos on the cover.

While looking over the haul he had set on one of the three rock piles, Charlie was startled by a crashing noise in the woods on the other side of the river. Instinctively, he ducked behind the rocks and looked in the direction of the crash. He sat unmoving for several minutes and never saw movement or heard a sound from the direction of the crash. *It was probably an animal. Maybe a deer or something*, he thought. He decided he had better get moving if he wanted to get back to his camper to get ready for the day. He was already cutting it close.

Charlie headed back the way he came, seeing nothing out of the ordinary or out of place. From behind him, on the other side of the stream, a man stepped out from behind a large tree to snap a few pictures with his phone and watch him leave.

. . .

When Charlie approached the clinic, he noticed the pickup truck parked in front. No minivan today; Dawn was back. He found Dave and Dawn both having coffee on the back patio. Dave waved him over and asked him to join them.

"Have some coffee, Charlie. You look tired," Dave said.

"I've been doing some hiking this morning," Charlie replied, deciding to keep his snooping and findings to himself. "Welcome back, Dawn. Everything okay in Marquette?"

After taking another sip of her coffee, she replied, "Yup. All good now. My dad needed some help, is all. He said it couldn't wait. Shouldn't be an issue now."

"Well, Charlie and I are glad to have you back, Dawn." Dave put a hand on her shoulder. "Just remember, if you need anything at all, don't hesitate to ask."

After Dave and Charlie filled Dawn in on what she had missed the day before, she politely excused herself to get the rooms ready for the day. Charlie and Dave discussed the PICO questions and answers that Charlie came up with for the previous day's cases.

Their first patient of the day didn't arrive until the clinic had been open an hour. Dave said that it went that way sometimes; some days were busy, while others were slow. He said they needed to use the slow days to their advantage, for studying and teaching.

Dawn let them know that their first patient was ready. It was another familiar face to start the day, Joseph Murphy.

. . .

Joseph R. Murphy's Neuropathy
Thursday, June 4
11:00 AM
Patient: Joseph R. Murphy
Age: 42

Charlie followed Dave into the room and stood against the wall to observe. Dave had indicated he was going to do the talking for this visit, and Charlie would jump in for the physical exam portion. Joe was in the clinic today to discuss a new concern. He had been dealing with some pain and numbness in his toes and feet, and it seemed to be getting worse.

"Good morning, Joe. Dawn tells me you're here because of your diabetic neuropathy. You've had signs of this before, so are you here because it's getting worse?" Dave asked.

"Oh, yeah. It's getting worse. It used to be only my toes were numb. Now I can't feel the bottom of my feet. And to make things worse, my feet hurt real bad now too."

"How do you mean?"

"Even though the bottom of my feet are numb, they hurt. It feels like I'm stepping on rocks all the time, and they tingle, kinda like they fell asleep. It's worse at night, and walking and standing all day at work don't help."

"How have your sugars been? Did you get the new insulin?" Dave asked.

"They haven't been too bad. It was 140 this morning. Had to pay a buttload for the insulin though. But if you say it's better than that stuff from the tribe, I'll do it. Ya know I trust ya, Doc."

> Diabetic neuropathy is one of the most common problematic complications of diabetes and leads to increased morbidity and mortality. It is responsible for ulcer formations and can lead to amputations. Routine screening and foot exams should be performed to attempt to recognize early symptoms. Improving glycemic control has been shown to slow the progression of most diabetic neuropathy, and among recently diagnosed or poorly controlled diabetics who show signs of new neuropathy, some may find symptoms reverse with tight glycemic control. However, studies on intensive glycemic control for chronic diabetic neuropathy are less promising (Vinik et al. 2013).

Dave had Charlie check out Joe's feet, do a heart and lung exam, and then review Joe's medication list out loud, mostly for Charlie's benefit. Dave discussed the reason it is important to continue monitoring his feet for cuts and injuries. With all the trail hiking, standing, and walking Joe does, he could put himself at risk for a pretty significant infection if he got a cut and didn't keep an eye on his feet. A serious infection could lead to an amputation. Joe said he was aware of the dangers. They also discussed treatment options for diabetic neuropathy. Dave reiterated that tight glycemic control is the best way to prevent worsening symptoms, and occasionally, well-controlled diabetes may actually improve symptoms. He made no promises of resolution, however.

As for pain relief, there were several options. Dave listed medications for nerve pain, specifically gabapentin and pregabalin, as well as antidepressants used for pain relief such as duloxetine, venlafaxine, amitriptyline, and nortriptyline. There are topical options as well, but Dave indicated that these were likely to be less effective, although cheaper.

"What about Norco, Doc?" Joe asked. "Some of the guys at work with this neuropathy pain take Norco. You think that would work?"

Dave shook his head and replied, "No. Although Norco works well for pain relief, this kind of pain is different. I don't think it's a good idea."

"You're the boss, Doc. I'll do whatever you suggest."

Changing the subject, Dave asked Joe if he'd been camping out on the trails lately.

"Why are you asking?" Joe replied, not giving a real answer to his question.

"Well, I came across a campsite recently that made me think of the time we camped on Grand Island and had trouble with that bear."

"Oh yeah? You see a campsite with bear scat all over?" Joe asked, grinning and nodding enthusiastically.

"No. No bear poop." Dave looked Joe in the eyes for a moment. "Beer cans strung on strings."

Joe's grin fell away. "No kidding?"

"Yeah," Dave replied solemnly. "Have you seen Able lately?"

"No. Heard he was around from some of the guys at the casino, but I haven't seen 'em."

"If you see him, tell him I need to talk to him, and remind him of 'leave no trace.' Can you do that for me, Joe?"

Joe nodded and got up to leave.

"Hold up a minute, Joe." Turning to Charlie, Dave said, "I need to speak with Joe about something privately. I'll be out in a minute, okay?"

Charlie nodded and stepped into the hall to wait for Dave so they could discuss treatment options for diabetic neuropathy.

ASSIGNMENT

Come up with a foreground (PICO) question based on this case. Find a study that answers your question, and appraise it for its Validity, Importance, and Usefulness. Use the worksheet in the appendix, and write a brief summary of the study, why you feel it answers your question adequately, and whether the study was valid, important, and useful in this case. What are some of the pros and cons of the study, and how will it impact the patient's care? What would you do after researching this question if you were the PA caring for this patient?

• • •

Max A. Garland and the Dog Bite
Thursday, June 4
11:30 AM
Patient: Max A. Garland
Age: 12

Dave and Charlie entered room one to see their last patient for the morning. They were seeing Max Garland, a twelve-year-old boy who was there with his father after being bitten by a dog. Dawn had warned them that the boy's hand looked pretty bad. She was planning on reviewing his shot records while they were in the room with the Garlands.

"Good morning. My name's Dave Harrington. I'm a PA here at the clinic, and this is Charlie. He's a PA student working with me today. Dawn tells me Max had a run-in with a dog. Is that right?" Dave asked as he sat down across from Mr. Garland at the small table against the wall. Charlie took up his post standing against the door to observe the conversation.

Max was sitting on the exam table and holding his right hand close to his chest. The hand was wrapped in a white T-shirt that was stained with blood. He looked surprisingly calm for someone in his position.

"Max tried to break up a scrum between our two dogs. Why don't you tell 'em what happened," Mr. Garland said, gesturing to Max.

"Benny and Nya were fighting over a deer antler. Nya started getting real mean with Benny so I tried to grab the antler while they were fighting. I thought maybe they'd stop fighting if there wasn't anything to fight over. But then she bit my hand when I grabbed it."

"Are Benny and Nya your dogs?" Dave asked.

"Yeah, Nya's a yellow lab, and Benny's a wiener dog mixed with something else. We don't really know what he's mixed with. They usually get along really well and only play fight," Max said.

"Nya has been known to be protective of her food or treats at times. I think she was just being protective of her antler. Max shouldn't have gone for the antler. He should have known better," Mr. Garland said.

"When Nya bit you, did she quickly bite and let go quickly? Or did she latch on longer?" Dave asked.

"It was real fast. I think she realized her mistake. After she bit me, she walked off with her tail between her legs," Max replied.

"Do your dogs have up-to-date vaccinations? Have they had their rabies shots?" Dave asked Mr. Garland.

"Yeah, they're all up-to-date."

"How about Max? Has he had all his childhood vaccinations? Are his vaccinations up-to-date as well?" Dave asked.

"I think so, but I don't see how that matters. Aren't we only worried about what the dog can give him and not the other way around?" Mr. Garland asked, looking a bit confused.

"Well, what's really important here is whether or not Max has received his tetanus shots. Animal bites, even from your own pets, are high-risk for transmitting tetanus. I'm sure he's protected if he's had his normal childhood vaccines, but we'll have Dawn look up his records on the online state registry to be sure."

Mr. Garland nodded as he understood. Dave stood up and walked over to the exam table and motioned Charlie to join him.

"Let's take a look at the bite, okay?" Dave said to Max.

Max slowly unwrapped his right hand and held it out for inspection. The bleeding had nearly stopped. The dog had bitten the right index finger and thumb.

There were puncture wounds noted on the thumb, but the finger looked much worse. The index finger wound was an open laceration. The skin was open with a flap, and a small amount of blood was weeping from the wound. Charlie didn't see any pulsations in the blood, so he suspected no arteries were damaged.

"Looks like she did a number on ya, didn't she?" Dave said to Max. Pointing for Charlie's benefit, he said, "If you look here, it looks like her bottom teeth punctured the thumb and snagged the index finger, causing the laceration. I'd say that goes along with his description of what happened. It doesn't look like the dog grabbed on or thrashed. The wound would have been much worse." He looked to Max and said, "I don't think she really meant to hurt you, Max. It looks like she was caught up in the moment."

Dave turned to Mr. Garland and let him know that they were going to get some supplies and come back to take care of the wound. They'd need to flush the wound first, and then he would write a prescription for antibiotics for Max.

In the hallway, Dave and Charlie discussed wound closures and animal bites. Some cases require leaving the wound partially opened to prevent further infection. They also discussed when antibiotics are needed and treatment options for Max.

ASSIGNMENT

Come up with a foreground (PICO) question based on this case. Find a study that answers your question, and appraise it for its Validity, Importance, and Usefulness. Use the worksheet in the appendix, and write a brief summary of the study, why you feel it answers your question adequately, and whether the study was valid, important, and useful in this case. What are some of the pros and cons of the study, and how will it impact the patient's care? What would you do after researching this question if you were the PA caring for this patient?

• • •

Melinda J. Hillard and the Question on Depression Treatment

Thursday, June 4

1:00 PM

Patient: Melinda J. Hillard

Age: 41

The first patient in the afternoon was Melinda Hillard, a woman who was suffering from depression. Dave again took the lead on this visit as he had a history with this patient.

"Hi, Mel. It's good to see you," Dave said, setting his papers on the desk to free his hands for a hug. Melinda and Dave hugged briefly, then they both sat down to talk.

"This is Charlie. He's a PA student here with me for a bit. Do you mind if he sits in on this visit?"

"No, that's fine," she replied. She looked sad. Her eyes barely looked up from the floor when she spoke. Her hands were clasped between her knees, and she rocked ever so slightly. She was wearing a baseball cap to cover unwashed hair, a pair of sweatpants, and a flannel top over a gray T-shirt. She looked like she hadn't slept well, as she had bags under her eyes.

"I heard about Mandy. I'm so sorry." Dave said as he placed his hands on hers.

Looking up to meet Dave's gaze, she replied, "I've known about her drug problems for a while now. We even tried to get her some help." She took some tissues and wiped away the tears that formed on her cheeks. "You hear about stuff like this all the time in the news, but you just don't think it'll happen to someone you love, you know?"

"Here." Dave gave her the box of tissues to hold. "Have you talked to anyone else about how you're feeling? Have you thought about counseling?"

"I haven't even left the house until today. Monty made me come in to see you. He says I can't get better by just lying around the house." More tears came with a burst of sobbing.

"Well, first, let me start by saying what you're feeling is perfectly normal. This is all part of grieving. We can't make the pain of losing your sister completely go away, but we can help you feel less lost; less overwhelmed. Successful treatment for something like this requires a lot of things. You need support—Monty, me, friends, family, we all support you. You don't have to go through this alone. Medications and counseling can help too."

"I don't know about medications, Dave. I don't want to rely on medication for the rest of my life."

"I don't want that for you either. I see medications like training wheels on a bike. They're there to help you feel more comfortable while you learn the skills needed to get better. After you master the skills needed, we can take the training wheels, or medication, away. The only way to do that in a timely manner is to learn the skills that come from counseling while on the medication."

Charlie listened and took notes while Dave counseled Melinda on techniques she could start to help with depression. Dave gave her names and numbers for counselors and grief counseling groups in the area. He suggested she start medication now, and after discussing different medication options, she was given a prescription to start. She was advised to follow up with him in about a month to see how things were going. He also advised her to call him on his cell if she needed anyone to talk to or felt unsafe. That surprised Charlie.

● ● ●

After she left, Charlie and Dave had time to sit in the office and discuss counseling techniques and medication options for depression. Dave filled Charlie in on who Melinda was.

"I've known Mel for several years now. She and I actually went on a few dates back when I first moved up here. She's married now to Monty Hillard. Monty runs a bait and tackle shop in Munising. We've stayed friends over the years. Mel's sister recently died from a drug overdose. She's the girl the fight at the Legion was over. She's the first drug overdose death in this area in years. Some folks around Munising think it was an isolated incident, while others think there's a drug problem brewing in town."

"What do you think?" Charlie asked.

"Oh, there's a drug problem all right, but I can't figure out where everyone is getting their drugs," Dave replied.

ASSIGNMENT

Come up with a foreground (PICO) question based on this case. Find a study that answers your question, and appraise it for its Validity, Importance, and Usefulness. Use the worksheet in the appendix, and write a brief summary of the study, why you feel it answers your question adequately, and whether the study was valid, important, and useful in this case. What are some of the pros and cons of the study, and how will it impact the patient's care? What would you do after researching this question if you were the PA caring for this patient?

• • •

Randy J. Ferguson and the Question on Blood Pressure Medications

Thursday, June 4

2:00 PM

Patient: Randy J. Ferguson

Age: 67

Later that afternoon, Dave sent Charlie into room three to see Randy Ferguson. According to Dawn, Randy was camping in the area and had forgotten his blood pressure medication at home. He was in to get refills on his medication.

Charlie entered the room and introduced himself before sitting down to take a medical history.

"So, Dawn tells us you're camping nearby, and you need a refill on your medications because you left them back home? Where's home?" Charlie asked as he pulled out his clipboard and pen.

"Downstate. My wife and I are from the Kalamazoo area. We come up here every summer for a few weeks. We like to do a little trail hiking, kayaking, and fishing. I love it up here. It's absolutely beautiful here. I guess we were in a bit of a hurry to get up here, and I forgot my medications. My wife used this facility when she twisted her ankle a few years back, and the service was wonderful so I figured I'd ask for your help."

"Well, I've only been here a few days, but I can certainly see what you mean about this place. I'm really enjoying my time here too. What medications did you leave at home?" Charlie asked.

"Luckily I only take a few medications and some supplements. I can get the supplements at the grocery store or pharmacy, but I'll need a prescription for my blood pressure meds. I take amlodipine and lisinopril," Randy replied.

"Do you happen to know the doses?" Charlie asked.

"Oh yeah, that's easy. Both are ten milligrams. I've been on the amlodipine for years, but my doc back home started me on the lisinopril about three months ago," Randy said.

Charlie consulted his notes from Dawn. Randy's blood pressure was elevated at 156/94, which was understandable considering that he wasn't on his medications.

"Well, your blood pressure is a little high. How long have you been without your medication?" Charlie asked.

"Only a few days. We left home on Monday."

"Have you had any symptoms related to the blood pressure? Any headaches, dizziness, or nosebleeds?" Charlie asked.

"No, none of that. I feel fine. Can't even tell the difference. Well, except my cough is gone," Randy said. "You think that could have anything to do with my blood pressure?"

Charlie thought about it for a moment and replied, "No, not directly, but your blood pressure medication could have been causing a cough. After you started taking the lisinopril, did you notice a new cough? Or was that there before starting the lisinopril?"

"Come to think of it, my cough did start a little while after starting the lisinopril. I never thought a medication could cause a cough. I always thought drug reactions were rashes and breathing trouble and such. You really think lisinopril could have caused my cough?" Randy asked.

Angiotensin-converting enzyme (ACE) inhibitors, like lisinopril, are routinely used to treat hypertension as they are quite effective in lowering blood pressure and are often very inexpensive. Like all medications, ACE inhibitors also have side effects, with a dry cough being one of the more common side effects experienced by 20 to 40 percent of patients. Studies suggest the increased release of bradykinin may be to blame. Alternatively, Angiotensin II receptor blockers (ARBs) don't seem to cause the cough as they work to lower blood pressure via blockade of the RAS system (Borghi and Veronesi, 2019).

"Well, the only way to be sure would be to put you back on it, but I'd suggest we just start you on something different. I need to talk to Dave first, but I'm pretty sure he'll want to start you back on amlodipine and probably a different medication to replace the lisinopril. Before we discuss that with him though, I'll need to get a little more information from you. Do you have any other heart disease or significant health issues?"

"No, I don't think so. What would you consider a significant health issue?" Randy asked.

"Oh, you know, diabetes, heart failure, high cholesterol, cancer. Anything like that?" Charlie asked.

"No, nothing too serious. My cholesterol was a little high at my last appointment, but I've been taking fish oil supplements and eating better, so I'm sure everything is good there."

"That's right. You said you were taking supplements. Other than the fish oil, what else do you take?"

"Oh, I take a baby aspirin, vitamin D3, licorice root, turmeric, and, of course, the fish oil," Randy said.

"Okay, I'll run these by Dave. Sometimes supplements can inadvertently raise your blood pressure as well. If we see any on the list that may raise your blood pressure, we'll let you know."

Charlie had Randy sit on the exam table as he performed a heart and lung exam, which was essentially normal. He also examined his head and neck, eyes, ears, nose, and throat. Everything checked out normal.

· · ·

When Charlie met up with Dave in the hallway and gave him a report on what he had found, they discussed blood pressure medications, side effects, alternatives for lisinopril, and how supplements may impact Randy's blood pressure. They also discussed what workup may or may not be needed for patients with hypertension.

They returned to the room together and discussed lifestyle modifications that could improve Randy's blood pressure and advised against taking licorice root. Then Dave gave him two prescriptions and asked him to return in a few weeks to see how his blood pressure was doing on the new regimen.

ASSIGNMENT

ASSIGNMENT

Come up with a foreground (PICO) question based on this case. Find a study that answers your question, and appraise it for its Validity, Importance, and Usefulness. Use the worksheet in the appendix, and write a brief summary of the study, why you feel it answers your question adequately, and whether the study was valid, important, and useful in this case. What are some of the pros and cons of the study, and how will it impact the patient's care? What would you do after researching this question if you were the PA caring for this patient?

. . .

Dave had to make a phone call, so Charlie was sent in to see Sarah Beedon, their next patient, who was in the office with some breathing trouble. Mrs. Beedon hadn't been to the clinic before, so there wasn't much information to go on prior to seeing her. All Dawn could decipher was that she had Chronic Obstructive Pulmonary Disease (COPD) and was still a smoker.

Sarah O. Beedon and the Case of COPD

Thursday, June 4

2:30 PM

Patient: Sarah O. Beedon

Age: 63

As Dave entered the room, Mrs. Beedon was seated in a chair and arranging her medications on the table next to her. The air smelled of stale cigarettes.

"Good afternoon, Mrs. Beedon. My name's Charlie. I'm a PA student working with Mr. Harrington. He'll be in to see you in a few minutes. He wanted me to come in and get some history from you and see how you're doing. Dawn says you're here because you're having some breathing difficulties?"

Mrs. Beedon stopped putting bottles on the table and looked up to Charlie and smiled. She looked much older than 63. There were wrinkles around her lips that Charlie thought must have been from years of smoking. She was thin with yellowed teeth and had a husky smoker's voice.

"That's right," she replied before slipping into a coughing fit. When she finished coughing, she took a few labored breaths and said, "It's my COPD. It's getting worse and my little red inhaler here doesn't seem to work as well as it used to." She waved what looked to Charlie to be an albuterol inhaler. "Although I suppose my smoking isn't helping," she said with a chuckle that triggered a cough.

"How long have you smoked?" Charlie asked.

"A long time. Maybe fifty years? I was just a young thing then," Mrs. Beedon said. "I've smoked about a pack a day since I was thirteen or so. It was the cool thing to do. I didn't get into any of the drugs back then, though. I just smoked."

"Have you ever thought about or tried quitting?" Charlie asked.

Mrs. Beedon laughed. "Honey, every smoker *thinks* about quitting smoking. Most just don't have the gumption to do it. I tried a few times to quit." She resumed putting bottles on the table. "I was able to go nine months without a cigarette when I was pregnant with my first daughter Linda, but I started up again soon after she was born. Too much stress, I guess." She put the last pill bottle on the table and leaned back in her chair. "There ya go. Here's all my meds. That lovely young nurse told me I could put them all up here so you can see what I take."

Charlie jotted down the names of several blood pressure medications, diabetes medications, antidepressants, and an inhaler. Mrs. Beedon was taking metformin and glipizide for diabetes, lisinopril and hydrochlorothiazide for hypertension, paroxetine for depression, and she had two different albuterol inhalers for COPD.

"Why do you have two albuterol inhalers?" Charlie asked.

"My doctor back home gave me that red one there, but I like the blue one because it's easier to use. I got it from an urgent care a few weeks ago. I'd like to get another one while I'm here if that's all right."

"I'm sure Dave would be willing to do that. So tell me about your trouble breathing. Is this new? How long have you been having trouble, like this, I mean." Charlie asked.

"Well, it doesn't take much for me to have a little trouble breathing. I've had some kind of trouble for years now. It's just been in the past couple years that I've had to take my inhalers every day. I used to only use them when I got a cold or something. Now every morning I wake up hacking with phlegm, and I get winded just walking to the mailbox. But that's been pretty normal for me the last few years. My doctor back home diagnosed me with COPD, gave me that albuterol, and told me to use it every day. He said he might have to add another inhaler if it didn't do enough. I guess that's why I'm here. I was hoping it would just get better and I could wait it out till I head back downstate in a few weeks, but I just can't wait anymore. It's exhausting not being able to breathe." Mrs. Beedon reached for her blue albuterol inhaler and took a puff.

"Have you had any fevers, chills, or cold-like symptoms?" Charlie asked.

"No, but I am pretty tired. I cough at night and wheeze. It keeps me from getting a good night's rest."

"I know you've heard it before, but if you quit smoking, it may help some. It'll at least slow the progression. Are you willing to try something to quit smoking while you are here?" Charlie asked.

Mrs. Beedon nodded. "I suppose I could give it a try. Just don't put me on those nicotine patches. They didn't work last time, and they cost too much money. If you have any other ideas, I'm game for hearing them," she replied.

"I'll talk it over with Dave to see what the best options are for you. First, let me take a listen to your lungs and see what's going on."

Charlie gestured for her to sit up on the exam table while he listened to her heart and lungs. Her heart sounded normal, but her lungs were not. She had diffuse wheezing with inspiration and expiration, and he could hear audible crackles in both upper lobes. The crackles cleared when she coughed. Charlie found no other abnormal findings on exam.

"Well, your lungs sound as one might expect for a smoker with COPD. Since Dave isn't back yet from his phone call, I'll go talk to him in the hall and we'll come back to let you know what we can do for you. Dave will likely prescribe another albuterol inhaler for you, but he may also put you on another inhaler for your COPD. We'll talk about what treatment options are best for smoking cessation, and we may get further testing to see how your lungs are working. Sit tight. I'll be back with Dave in a few minutes."

As Charlie closed the door behind him, Dave came out of his office and started to the exam room.

"Did I miss it all?" Dave asked. "What do we have?"

"The patient is Mrs. Beedon, a sixty-three-year-old with COPD. She has a fifty-year history of smoking a pack a day and has COPD. She only uses albuterol, but it isn't working anymore. Basically, we need to get her COPD under control and help her quit smoking. She says she is ready; she just doesn't want to use patches," Charlie reported.

Dave and Charlie discussed COPD treatment options as well as options for medications to assist in smoking cessation. Dave suggested Charlie should do further research with a PICO question on these as well.

They returned to the room and informed Mrs. Beedon of their decision: she was to get a pulmonary function test and a chest x-ray.

In the hall as they watched Mrs. Beedon leave, Dave clapped Charlie on the shoulder and said, "Nice work, Charlie, nice work."

ASSIGNMENT

Come up with a foreground (PICO) question based on this case. Find a study that answers your question, and appraise it for its Validity, Importance, and Usefulness. Use the worksheet in the appendix, and write a brief summary of the study, why you feel it answers your question adequately, and whether the study was valid, important, and useful in this case. What are some of the pros and cons of the study, and how will it impact the patient's care? What would you do after researching this question if you were the PA caring for this patient?

• • •

Later that afternoon, Charlie was sent to talk to Dustin Tebear, who reported his chief complaint as substance abuse. Dustin stated that he had been using Norco and Percocet to get high for the past few months and wanted help to quit. After his conversation with Dave earlier, Charlie was starting to think the local drug problem wasn't brewing, but actually boiling over.

"Good afternoon. My name is Charlie. I'm a PA student working with Dave. I'll be taking care of you today. Dave will be in shortly as well. What can I do for you?"

"Charlie, I think I've got a problem. In fact, I know I have a problem." Rocking a little with his right knee bouncing rapidly, Dustin shook his head. "I did something stupid, man. I started taking some painkillers at work for my back, and before I knew it, I started taking them like candy all day long. There's this guy at work who sells the stuff. He gave me a few to try when I tweaked my back. I didn't think it'd be that big of a deal. He said they'd help, and they did a little. But then he offered to sell me something a little stronger. He said it would help me sleep."

"What did you take?" asked Charlie.

Dustin, still fidgeting, wiped sweat off his brow. "Norco. Now I'm on Percocets."

"How many do you take in a day?"

"I take like eight throughout the day. Something like that. I don't know, man. I don't really count them. I tried to go without, but when I do, I want to throw up, I get achy all over, I sweat a lot, and I can't sleep. I don't want to keep taking them, man, but I don't want to die from withdrawal either!"

"Well, for starters, you can't die from opioid withdrawals, but you might feel like you'd want to. How long is the longest you've gone without a pill?"

"I took one last night before bed. I didn't take any today yet, and it's killing me, man!"

"All right, let me take a look at you and then get Dave in here to talk to you too. Then we'll see what we can do for the withdrawal symptoms."

Charlie listened to his heart and lungs, checked out his abdomen, and examined his skin for track marks. He found no evidence of intravenous drug use, and other than his clammy, sweaty skin, the remaining exams were normal. When Dave came in, he repeated the exams and discussed opioid withdrawals, addiction issues, and treatment options. They talked about weaning, stopping "cold turkey," and using medications like buprenorphine/naloxone or methadone. Dave gave him a prescription and provided him with a pamphlet that had the names, addresses, and phone numbers for various local addiction help centers.

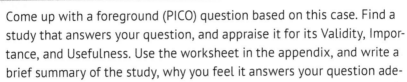

ASSIGNMENT

Come up with a foreground (PICO) question based on this case. Find a study that answers your question, and appraise it for its Validity, Importance, and Usefulness. Use the worksheet in the appendix, and write a brief summary of the study, why you feel it answers your question adequately, and whether the study was valid, important, and useful in this case. What are some of the pros and cons of the study, and how will it impact the patient's care? What would you do after researching this question if you were the PA caring for this patient?

$\bullet \quad \bullet \quad \bullet$

Paddling for Therapy

After the clinic closed for the day, Charlie went back to his camper to get ready for an overnight kayaking excursion. The office was closed on Friday mornings, reopening in the afternoon. To make up for lost time on Fridays, the clinic was open Saturday mornings until noon. Dave had invited Charlie to come along on an overnight campout on Grand Island. They were to kayak out to the island, make camp on the western shore, and be back by lunchtime Friday. Charlie was genuinely excited to go on this short trip. Before arriving for rotation, he had researched the area and made a bucket list of things to do as time allowed. Trips to check out the trails and waterways around Munising topped his list. Grand Island and Pictured Rocks were underlined and circled on his list.

Charlie grabbed a change of clothes, his hoodie sweatshirt, and a pair of jeans and threw them in his backpack. He reached for his phone, hesitated, and then decided to bring it for pictures.

He waited at the front entrance of the campground for a short while before Dave's Jeep pulled up. The top was down, and a passenger sat in the front seat.

"Hop in, Charlie!" As Charlie climbed over the side of the Jeep into the back seat, Dave introduced his passenger. "Charlie, this is Ryan. Ryan, this is Charlie."

"Nice to meet you," Charlie said to Ryan. He reached out and shook his hand before settling in the back seat.

Ryan looked a little distracted to Charlie. He had briefly looked to Charlie with a half-hearted smile when they shook hands, but then he returned his gaze out the side window. He didn't say much on their way to the kayak launch.

Earlier, when Dave had invited Charlie on this excursion, he told him they would be bringing Ryan along. He explained that Ryan was the young man who had gotten into the fight at the American Legion. Mandy, the girl who had unfortunately overdosed, had been Ryan's girlfriend. Like Mandy, Ryan had dabbled in drugs, mostly opioids on a recreational basis. When Mandy overdosed and died, he took it pretty hard. Dave had taken Ryan under his wing after he learned of the tragic accident. Ryan was the one Dave met for dinner on Monday, and Ryan was the guest who came by the office on Tuesday asking for help. This trip was part of what Dave called ecotherapy. He said some psychologists call it nature therapy or green therapy. Physical activity in nature and meditation are two of the most useful aspects of ecotherapy. Obviously, the kayaking was the physical activity in mind with this trip. He further explained that the kayaking would provide Ryan with increased awareness of the natural world and help reduce his depression and anger. They would work on meditation that evening at sunset to help fight his depressed mood.

When they reached the Grand Island Ferry dock, which happened to have a kayak launch as well, Charlie wasn't surprised to see Joseph standing by a pickup truck with a trailer full of kayaks behind it. He was waving them over to his truck. Dave parked his Jeep, and they all climbed out and helped unload the kayaks. Joseph had brought four single-person tents and blankets for them to use. They piled their luggage into the kayaks and headed out across the channel to William's Landing on the southernmost point of Grand Island.

They paddled across the channel and then headed west along the coast. Joseph led the way a few kayak lengths ahead of the group, while Dave brought up the rear. Charlie found himself alongside Ryan after they made the bend around Merchandise Beach, about a mile from William's Landing. They were now on the west coast of the island and making their way north. Charlie noticed that Ryan looked more focused and less distracted now that he was breaking a sweat paddling along the shoreline.

"You ever kayak around here before?" Charlie asked.

"Around Grand Island? No. I've done lots of kayaking in smaller lakes and rivers, but I've never been out on Superior in a kayak before," Ryan replied, finally making meaningful eye contact with Charlie for the first time that night.

Charlie thought he looked like he was getting better already. Maybe this ecotherapy had some merit after all. Ryan's cheeks were flushed from exercise, and his eyes, formerly downcast and dull, seemed to appear clearer.

"Not sure why either. I've lived in the U.P. my whole life, and I've never even been on a Pictured Rocks tour or anything like that," Ryan said, returning his eyes to the front of his kayak.

"You like camping?" Charlie asked.

"Yeah, sure. I've been camping lots. I wasn't really sure about coming out tonight, but Dave can be pretty persuasive. He's a good dude." Ryan paused his paddling and coasted for a moment. When he started paddling again, he looked to Charlie. "You're pretty lucky to have him as a teacher. We need more docs like Dave. He really cares about people, you know?"

Charlie did know. He was seeing that Dave really put himself out there often.

• • •

They had paddled for about two and a half hours since leaving the dock on the mainland, covering about three and a half miles or so. Joseph gestured for the group to head to the shore. They beached the kayaks and tied them to a tree on the beach, then hiked with their gear up a short path to a campsite overlooking the lakefront.

After setting up camp, Joseph started bringing large stones up from the shore. Dave explained to Ryan and Charlie that these stones would be used as part of the meditation portion of the trip. With the sun setting over the water and the sound of the waves crashing on the shore below, Dave and Joseph worked with Ryan on meditation and counseling. They slowly stacked the rocks in formations around the campsite "to ward off negative thoughts." Charlie watched this with an understanding. He recognized the stacked rocks as the same setup he had seen at the abandoned campsite the Scouts found. Dave had said he'd seen a site like that before, and now Charlie wondered if Dave knew more about the site than he was letting on.

When Dave, Joseph, and Ryan finished with meditation, the sun was getting low on the water and darkness was creeping on.

"We'd better get a bear bag up, eh? Don't want to find our breakfast gone and bear scat everywhere in the morning," Joseph remarked with a grin. He gathered the food and hoisted it in a bag on a high branch several yards away from the campsite.

Bear scat, Charlie mused, thinking of the conversation with Joseph earlier that day in the office. Dave and Joseph had talked about camping on the island in the past, and Joseph had joked about bear scat. Dave had redirected the questioning to beer cans strung on string. There were no cans on string here tonight.

"Is the rock stacking a technique of meditation commonly used in ecotherapy?" Charlie asked Dave.

"Well, meditation can be done in a number of ways. The rock stacking is actually something Joseph taught me years ago."

"I learned it from Noos," chimed in Joseph.

"Noos?"

"*Noos* means 'my father' in Ojibwa. He taught me and my brother when we were young. 'To have peace of mind and ward off bad dreams, stack three piles of rocks around your campsite' Noos used to say. When stacked in meditation, you ward off negative stuff," Joseph said while starting a fire.

"Is that still fairly common?" Charlie asked, thinking of the abandoned site.

"Nah. Only people I ever known to do it is me, Noos, and ..." Joseph trailed off and looked to Dave. Dave met his glance and then turned to look out to the water.

The sun had sunk below the water, leaving only a pink water-colored smear across the darkening sky.

"Soak it in, guys. The sky up here at night is gorgeous. Don't stay up too late though. We gotta break camp and get moving pretty early if we want to be back to the dock by 11 a.m. Still gotta work tomorrow," Dave said. He leaned back against a tree with his arms behind his head and stared off over the water.

Ryan poked the fire with a stick. It looked to Charlie like the trip had been good for Ryan, but there was still a melancholy about him.

Feeling tired, Charlie climbed into his tent to call it a night. He looked out through the screen window at the stars above and soon drifted off to sleep.

CHAPTER 5

Friday

Morning Revelations

Charlie pulled the edge of his sleeping bag over his head to block out the crisp, cool air of morning. He didn't want to get up and moving, but his bladder offered a fairly convincing rebuttal. Resentfully, he unzipped the tent, got out, and made his way to a fairly private collection of shrubbery to relieve himself.

As per his usual routine, he was up fairly early. Old habits die hard he supposed. No matter how tired he was or late he stayed up, he always seemed to be a morning person. You could set your watch to it. Sure enough, Charlie's watch read 6:04 a.m. When he returned to his tent, he wasn't surprised to find snores coming from Ryan's tent next to his. He didn't hear anything coming from Dave's or Joseph's tent either. Charlie grabbed his gear and repacked his bag. He put on his hoodie and jeans for the cool paddle back to the dock. It was pretty chilly, and the air over the cold lake wouldn't do much to warm him this morning. He wished they would have brought a way to make coffee.

With his tent taken down and his bag packed, Charlie decided to enjoy the view of the lake while he waited for the others to get up. He made his way to the cliff edge by the beach, intending to sit and watch the waves. He heard voices so he stopped and crouched to listen, not wanting to be seen. It sounded like Dave and Joseph. Had they been out of their tents all this time? As he slowly approached the edge, he could see Dave and Joseph talking down by the kayaks.

"Why didn't you tell me he was back from Chicago?" Dave asked.

"I didn't know till this week, I swear. I thought he still had a couple years left till probation. I haven't even seen him yet. Some brother he is. Doesn't even say 'hey' to his own flesh and blood when he gets back to town."

"Did you check out the campsite I told you about? It's gotta be his. Didn't look like it was used in a while though."

"Yeah, it'd be his all right. He must be spooked or something. Why else would he use the cans, heh? You think someone's out to get him or something?"

"Maybe. Or maybe he's up to no good. Why else would he be camping in the woods? Why not call you up and stay with you? Seems suspicious."

"Yeah, well, he might have called someone else besides me."

"Like an old girlfriend or something." Dave nodded. He checked his wrist and said, "Better get back. We need to ship out soon to make it back at a reasonable time."

Charlie backed away from the ledge and stood. He casually walked to the edge and pretended to see Dave and Joseph for the first time.

"Morning, guys! I'm not the only early riser, I see," Charlie called out, waving. "I was looking for you guys. I saw you weren't in your tents. I was wondering where you hung the bear bag. You don't happen to have a coffee maker in there, do you?" he said with a smirk while holding up both hands with crossed fingers.

As it turned out, Joseph did bring a coffeepot with some coffee and a Jetboil.

• • •

The four of them cleared out of camp and paddled back to the ferry dock. The overcast morning was cool, and the water was cold. With a little northernly wind to their backs they were able to make pretty good time in the kayaks. Nobody said much. When they reached the dock, Ryan shook each of their hands and thanked them for the evening. He said he would be back the next day for a follow-up appointment at the clinic to discuss his mood.

Charlie had about an hour and a half to shower, eat, change, and be ready for the afternoon at the clinic. He jotted some notes down about ecotherapy and studied what he could find. He enjoyed his trip to the island but was happy to get back to seeing patients again in the clinic. He hoped he'd see some interesting cases today.

• • •

The clinic opened at 1 p.m. on Friday afternoons. When Charlie walked over to the clinic at 12:30 p.m., Dawn was already there. Dave hadn't gotten there yet. Charlie told Dawn about their trip and filled her in on what he had heard. She seemed interested in all of it, until he mentioned Joseph having a brother who was seemingly out of prison early. She quickly changed the subject back to Ryan and told Charlie what she knew about Mandy's overdose. Apparently, Mandy had been at a party with Ryan and was offered fentanyl instead of her usual Percocet from a dealer. She overdosed at the party, and Ryan was trying to pick a fight with the guy who sold it to her when he saw him at the American Legion the other day. Dawn said that rumors around town indicated the drugs in the area were coming from a big city dealer who was using a local to get them out.

When Dave came in, the conversation about Ryan and Mandy stopped. Dave and Charlie reviewed the schedule for the day and discussed cases that Dave thought Charlie could take the lead on. The first scheduled appointment for the day looked like a great fit for Charlie. He'd see a familiar face as Jason Varney was back for more burn debridement and to discuss a rash.

•   •   •

Charlie entered room one and greeted Jason Varney. The last time Mr. Varney was in the office, he was complaining of some back pain along with getting his burn debridement. It was a bit awkward for Charlie during that visit as Mr. Varney and Dave had butted heads over a prescription for Norco. Dave had stuck to his guns, and Mr. Varney had left with only the suggestion of taking naproxen.

Jason K. Varney and His Rash
Friday, June 5
1:30 PM
Patient: Jason K. Varney
Age: 37

"Good afternoon, kid. How's the rotation going for ya?" Jason asked. He was seated on the exam table with his arms crossed across his chest.

"It's going well, thanks. I'm learning a lot, and I've been able to see a lot of the surrounding area as well," Charlie replied. "How's the hand?"

"It's good. Pretty much healed I'd say. Mr. Harrington wanted me to come in for a recheck if I were still here today, so here I am. I don't think anything needs to be done for it. I do have another reason for being here though. Two reasons actually. I know you can probably help me with one, and maybe you can help me with the other."

"Well, let's look at the hand first and see how it looks," Charlie said.

Charlie unwrapped the lightly wrapped left hand to find scarring, but no open flesh anymore. His wound had healed nicely. Mr. Varney was correct in his own assessment; no more treatment was needed.

"Congratulations, Mr. Varney, your hand looks great! That healed pretty fast!"

"One of the other reasons I'm here today is that I've got this rash on my right shin. I've had it for years, and I used to have a cream for it, but I forgot it at home when I packed to come up here on my hike. The rash itches and drives me nuts. I used some over-the-counter hydrocortisone cream I had in my pack, and it helped some but isn't going away."

"How long have you had the rash?" Charlie asked.

"Years."

Charlie asked to take a peek, and Jason pulled up his right pant leg. There was a raised, red, scaly patch of psoriasis about the size of a deck of cards on his right shin. The skin around it was erythematous. *A classic case of psoriasis,* Charlie thought.

"Looks like you have psoriasis."

"Yeah, I know," Jason interrupted. "I know what it is. I just wanted something better for the itch than the hydrocortisone cream I got."

"Do you remember what you were treated with before? Did it work okay?"

"No, I don't remember the name of the stuff, but it was an ointment. A steroid I'm sure. I've been on a few different creams and ointments over the years. I'd be open to trying something different if you have any ideas."

"Okay, well, I'm sure we can certainly get you a prescription for a steroid ointment, or if Dave thinks something else would be better, maybe we could clear it up and keep it gone. I'll just talk to Dave about the options for psoriasis treatment and see what we can get you." Charlie stood up and started to head to the door to get Dave.

"Hold up, kid. There's one more thing I'd like to talk to you about. Just you. It's important."

Charlie stopped before opening the door and looked back to Jason.

"Sit down. Please." Jason reached into his back pocket and pulled out something to show Charlie. He looked amused at seeing the confusion and bewilderment on Charlie's face when he saw the badge.

ASSIGNMENT

Come up with a foreground (PICO) question based on this case. Find a study that answers your question, and appraise it for its Validity, Importance, and Usefulness. Use the worksheet in the appendix, and write a brief summary of the study, why you feel it answers your question adequately, and whether the study was valid, important, and useful in this case. What are some of the pros and cons of the study, and how will it impact the patient's care? What would you do after researching this question if you were the PA caring for this patient?

• • •

Tabitha A. Bonkowski and the Case of Asthma

Friday, June 5

2:00 PM

Patient: Tabitha A. Bonkowski

Age: 28

Charlie was relieved when Dave suggested they go together to see their next patient, Tabby Bonkowski. He had a lot to think about after talking with Mr. Varney, or Officer Varney? He didn't know what to call him. Either way, he needed time to think and was grateful for the opportunity to fade back into the shadows and let Dave do the talking with this patient.

Tabby was there to get a refill on her albuterol inhaler for her asthma. She was seated on the exam table and texting away on her phone when they entered the room. She looked up and smiled when she saw Dave.

"Hey, Dave! Oh my God, I'm so glad I was able to get this appointment today. I gotta be to work in like thirty minutes. I thought I had an extra inhaler in my car, but it was empty. I need another albuterol inhaler. I'm all out, and with my weekend shift starting today and all those smokers at the casino, I'm really gonna need one. Can ya help a girl out?" she rapidly spit out.

"Whoa, slow down. You need another albuterol inhaler? How often do you use your inhaler?" Dave asked.

"Like, only four or five times a day. I definitely use it more often at work. Those smokers get my asthma going every time, but the tips are totally worth it," she said.

"Are you using it because you have trouble breathing or is it because you're wheezing?" Dave asked.

"Both, I guess. Sometimes I wheeze, but other times it's just my chest feels tight. It's not so bad when I'm working around the slots, but lately I've been working the poker room, and there's usually a cloud of smoke in that room."

Dave nodded. "You're not smoking too, are you?"

"What, like cigarettes? No way. I stay away from that stuff. Smoking is like totally bad for you if you've got asthma."

"So is working around so much smoke," Dave replied, raising an eyebrow.

"I know, I know. But the money is good. Do you have any idea how hard it is to find a job that pays good around here? At least I'm not selling drugs or nothin'."

Charlie was suddenly more interested in this conversation.

"Do people sell drugs at the casino?" Charlie asked.

Dave looked back to Charlie, a little puzzled. "I don't ... see how that is relevant here?" Looking back to Tabby, he asked, "Are you taking any other medications for your asthma?"

Ignoring Dave's question, Tabby replied to Charlie. "Sure, it's a casino. There are people who sell drugs, mostly pot or pain pills." She returned her gaze to Dave. "But I don't do any of that stuff," she said, smiling. "And no. All I've got for asthma is my albuterol."

"Well, if you're unwilling to change your environment, which I would strongly suggest as it's likely making your asthma worse, and you're using your albuterol all the time, I'd suggest we add a maintenance inhaler so you won't need the albuterol all the time."

"You see, your albuterol inhaler should be considered your emergency inhaler. If you're having an emergency several times a day, most days, you really should be using an all-day inhaler that will keep your airways open longer. If you haven't been on anything before, I'd suggest adding a low-dose inhaled corticosteroid inhaler," Dave said.

"I'll send a prescription for one, along with a refill on your albuterol, to your pharmacy. Would you mind coming back in a week or two to do a pulmonary function test?" Dave asked.

"Sure, I can do that, but I really do need to get to work. I'll call back later to set up the follow-up appointment," she said.

"Great. Why don't I take a listen to your heart and lungs before I step out to send the prescriptions in?" Dave said.

After they left the room, Dave pulled Charlie aside. They talked about asthma treatments and testing. Charlie asked how to choose between different medications in the same class. Which were better? Dave suggested he look into it later for a research topic.

Charlie was surprised Dave didn't mention his question about drugs. He didn't know whether he should be relieved or worried that Dave didn't want to talk about it.

ASSIGNMENT

Come up with a foreground (PICO) question based on this case. Find a study that answers your question, and appraise it for its Validity, Importance, and Usefulness. Use the worksheet in the appendix, and write a brief summary of the study, why you feel it answers your question adequately, and whether the study was valid, important, and useful in this case. What are some of the pros and cons of the study, and how will it impact the patient's care? What would you do after researching this question if you were the PA caring for this patient?

• • •

Garrett D. Bazany Was Scratched by a Bat

Friday, June 5

2:30 PM

Patient: Garrett D. Bazany

Age: 27

For the next appointment that afternoon, Charlie again accompanied Dave, who did most of the talking. They were seeing Garrett Bazany, a twenty-seven-year-old who was visiting the area with a few college friends. He was in the office because he believed he had been bitten by a bat the night before.

As they entered the room, Garrett was seated in a wheelchair next to the exam table and holding what looked like a torn piece of clothing around his left thigh. Seated in the chair by the desk was a bored-looking young woman. Her eyes never left her cell phone, even as Dave introduced himself.

"Good afternoon! My name's Dave. I'm a PA, and this is Charlie. He's a student working with me for the next few months. Dawn tells me you're here today because you were bitten by a bat? How'd that happen?"

"I'm actually not a hundred percent sure I was bitten. Last night there was a bat in our cabin, and after we finally were able to shoo it outside, I noticed my left leg had been cut. My friends were swatting it with a broom, and at one point, the bat had fluttered in my hair and landed on my lap. I don't know if it bit me or not, so I wanted to get checked out. I don't want rabies or anything," Garrett said.

"Hold on. Let's go back to the bat in the cabin story. When did this happen?" Dave asked.

"Last night we were all playing cards and drinking in our cabin," Garrett started.

"We're on a couples retreat with a few other couples from school," the girl added, without looking away from her phone.

"We're all up here to do some kayaking, biking, and enjoying outdoor stuff," Garrett said. He must have seen Charlie's eyebrows go up because he added, "I may be in a wheelchair, but I still know how to have a good time."

At this comment the girl looked up from her phone and said, "He's like a pro on his handcycle mountain bike. With sponsors and everything."

"So ... last night you were all playing cards ..." Dave said.

"Right. We were all playing cards, and my buddy Ian came back from a beer run and accidentally let a bat in when he left the door open for too long. It was flying all around the room, and Rachel here thought it'd be a good idea to take the broom from the closet and try to kill it or something."

"I wasn't trying to kill it; I was just trying to stun it so we could throw it outside or something, I swear!" Rachel said.

"Whatever. So, she hit the bat, but it didn't get stunned or die or anything. It landed in my lap, and when I tried to throw it off with my hands, it flew up and got in my hair. It then fluttered to the window and hit the window."

"That knocked it out. Go figure," Rachel said.

"Yeah, then Ian tossed it outside," Garrett said.

"You said you think it may have bitten you, but you aren't sure? Couldn't you feel it if it bit you?" Charlie asked.

"Nah, I don't really have much feeling in my legs. I had a fracture at C7 when I was a teenager so I don't really have much feeling from the waist down."

"Well, let's take a look," Dave said.

Garrett moved the torn cloth off the left upper leg to reveal several scratches that didn't seem too deep. There was no sign of infection, and no need for sutures.

"Looks like you were scratched, not bitten. We'll clean this up and get you the post-exposure prophylaxis treatment. Have you ever received a rabies vaccine before?" Dave asked.

"No."

"Okay, so in this case, I'll have Dawn give you two shots. You'll get a rabies immune globulin shot and a rabies vaccine. You'll need to come back for some subsequent shots throughout the week. Dawn will fill you in on that," Dave said.

After cleaning Garrett's wounds under Dave's supervision, Charlie bandaged the wounds, and together they stepped out to let Dawn give the shots.

Back in the hallway, Charlie asked Dave a number of questions about rabies and treatments. He wanted to know when and how to treat for rabies. Dave suggested he do some research and get back to him the next day on the topic.

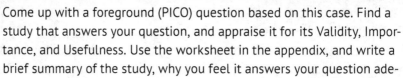

ASSIGNMENT

Come up with a foreground (PICO) question based on this case. Find a study that answers your question, and appraise it for its Validity, Importance, and Usefulness. Use the worksheet in the appendix, and write a brief summary of the study, why you feel it answers your question adequately, and whether the study was valid, important, and useful in this case. What are some of the pros and cons of the study, and how will it impact the patient's care? What would you do after researching this question if you were the PA caring for this patient?

· · ·

Scott C. Halliday Has an Itchy Rash

Friday, June 5

3:00 PM

Patient: Scott C. Halliday

Age: 14

Later that afternoon, Charlie found himself seeing another group of familiar faces. The Scout troop that had been camping nearby this week was in the office again, this time for a case of poison ivy rash. Because Charlie had developed a good relationship with many of the Scouts, Dave decided to send him in alone first, to get a history and examine the rash.

"I'd like to say that I'm surprised to see you guys here again, but you seem to be making this a habit," Charlie greeted the Scouts with a smile.

"We can't seem to stay away!" replied the Scout leader.

Seated on the exam table was Scott Halliday, a fourteen-year-old Scout with a rash on his arms and legs. The rest of the boys leaned against the wall and looked very disinterested.

"Are we all better from our diarrhea?" he asked Gage, who was practicing knot tying with some scrap rope as he leaned against the wall. "How about your foot?" he asked Robbie, who stood next to Gage.

"All better," they both replied.

Charlie directed his attention to Scott. "Looks like you've gotten into some poison ivy. When did you first notice the rash?"

"Last night my legs and arms started itching pretty bad. I thought it was from mosquito bites or something. When I woke up this morning, I found red blistery looking lines on my legs and arms," replied Scott, absently rubbing his left upper arm.

"Stop itching, Scott" said the tallest Scout standing against the wall.

"I know, Ben!" he replied, still rubbing his arm.

"Have you been walking through the woods off the trail?" Charlie asked.

"Yeah, we played capture the flag not too far from our campsite Wednesday night. Ben found the poison ivy near where we were playing. I only wore shorts and a T-shirt. The other guys wore dark pants and long sleeves to be better camouflaged. We must have gone through the poison ivy patch."

"I can confirm the poison ivy," said the Scout leader. "We've been pointing it out along the trail, but I suppose it would be hard to find in the dark without a flashlight."

"Well, the rash seems to be pretty extensive. I could give you a topical cream for it, or perhaps some oral steroids. A shot may be in order as well, but I'll have to talk to Dave about it. For future reference, if you think you might have gotten in some poison ivy, the best thing to do is to wash the area or shower with soap and water as soon as possible after exposure. Studies have shown that even washing the oils of the plant off up to two hours later can be effective. Maybe you guys should wash up after playing?"

Patients will often reach for over-the-counter remedies to treat the itch associated with their contact dermatitis from poison ivy. There are several products available for purchase that claim to effectively wash away the urushiol or oil that causes the allergic reaction. Other agents, such as topical antihistamines or topical antipruritics (like calamine) are commonly used to relieve itching.

There are several natural remedies that patients have been known to reach for as well. Jewelweed sap has been used to treat various rashes, including poison ivy. Witch hazel, baking soda paste, and apple cider vinegar have all been tried as natural remedies as well.

Why do providers need to know about these options? Perhaps your patient won't be able to afford prescription treatments, can't come into a clinic, or may have other barriers to treatment. Education for patients and providers alike on alternative treatments is vital to providing adequate care. I would encourage you to look into the research available on these treatments and provide information on useful "natural" treatments whenever possible.

"We'll take whatever treatment you can give us. We're starting our hike back to Tahquamenon Falls tomorrow afternoon. We're so glad there was an urgent care here by the campground since we needed to use it so much while we were here. Thanks for everything," the Scout leader said.

"Before I head out to get Dave, can I ask you guys something?" Charlie asked.

"Sure. What's up?" replied the Scout leader.

"Do you guys remember that abandoned campsite you found? Are you guys heading back that way by chance?"

"No, sorry. We aren't headed that way anymore. We'll be heading south on the Pipeline and then east to the North Country Trail. Why?"

"Just wondering," Charlie replied. After a moment of thought he added, "If you guys see anything weird or suspicious out there on the Pipeline or around the campgrounds today, could you let me know?"

"Sure, I suppose we could do that. How do we get ahold of you?"

"Here's my cell number," Charlie replied. He wrote his number on the back of a patient education sheet on plants to avoid on the trails. "If I don't answer, leave a message. Or you could just text me too if that's easier."

"Will do," said the Scout leader. He folded the paper and put it in his back pocket.

* * *

Charlie left the room and found Dave in his office on the phone. He looked agitated and not at all happy with whomever was on the other end of the line. After a minute or two, he hung up and looked up to Charlie.

"All done in there? What have they gotten themselves into this time?" he asked Charlie.

"Poison ivy dermatitis. Just one boy, though. It's pretty extensive on his arms and legs. I wasn't sure if you'd only treat with topical steroids, use oral or a shot, or some combination."

They discussed treatment options and went in together to let the boy know what the plan was.

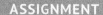
ASSIGNMENT

Come up with a foreground (PICO) question based on this case. Find a study that answers your question, and appraise it for its Validity, Importance, and Usefulness. Use the worksheet in the appendix, and write a brief summary of the study, why you feel it answers your question adequately, and whether the study was valid, important, and useful in this case. What are some of the pros and cons of the study, and how will it impact the patient's care? What would you do after researching this question if you were the PA caring for this patient?

* * *

Dave sent Charlie in to see Ms. Gerry Robertson at 4 p.m. She was in the office to get a refill on her acyclovir for cold sores. Before he entered the room, Dawn filled Charlie in on some background info regarding Ms. Robertson. Gerry lived in Munising and was a retired grocery store clerk in town. Her husband was Dr. Robertson, the medical director for the clinic. According to Dawn, Dr. Robertson has Gerry use the clinic for refills as a way of keeping an eye on the clinic.

Gerry Robertson and the Question on Treating Cold Sores
Friday, June 5
4:00 PM
Patient: Gerry Robertson
Age: 75

The fact that Dave was sending Charlie in alone spoke volumes to his confidence in his student's ability.

Charlie entered the room and introduced himself to the well-dressed elderly woman seated on the exam table.

"Good afternoon, Ms. Robertson. My name is Charlie, and I'm a PA student working with Dave Harrington for a couple months. I'll be taking a history and doing a quick exam before Dave comes in to wrap up the visit. Dawn tells me you're here today for a refill on your acyclovir. Is that correct?"

"That's right. I use it for cold sores I get from time to time on my lower lip here," she said, pointing to a dark spot on the right side of her lower lip. "I've had cold sores off and on for years. It usually pops up if I get sick or if I'm stressed. When that happens, I just take some of my acyclovir pills, and it usually takes care of it."

"Have you been feeling ill lately?" Charlie asked.

"Oh no, nothing like that, dear. I've just been a little more stressed than usual. That's all. This outbreak started a few days ago with some tingling, and as you can see, it is starting to blister some."

"Have you ever taken the medication daily instead of episodically? Or perhaps, have you tried other medication options like topical medication?" Charlie asked.

"I've been on the same regimen for years. My husband put me on this medication and instructs me how to take it. I just need refills today is all. It works just fine by me."

"Well, if you don't mind me asking, what's gotten your stress up lately?" Charlie asked.

Ms. Robertson took a deep breath, sighed, and got off the exam table. She walked over to the chair by the wall and started looking through her purse. When she found what she was looking for, she handed it to Charlie.

Charlie held a prescription bottle that was empty and void of any label.

"I don't understand." Charlie said.

"No, I don't suppose you would. That bottle was taken from my grandson's bedroom last week. The bottle had pills inside before my husband disposed of them. He says they looked like prescription pain pills. We spoke with my son and his wife, and they were going to talk to my grandson." She held her hand out and took the bottle back from Charlie.

"The clinic just opened for the season this week, so I suppose you've only been in town a short while. You may not have heard this yet, but there is a bit of a drug problem brewing in our little town, has been for a few years now, I'd say. Rest assured, this issue doesn't really reflect on the folks who live and work here. They're all good, hardworking people. My husband suspects the drugs are coming in from an outside source because he doesn't think it could be coming from the clinic. He doesn't think Dave is that kind of provider."

Charlie nodded. He thought highly of Dave too. Perhaps this information would be good to share with Officer Varney.

Thinking he'd better get things back on track with regards to her office visit, Charlie asked her to sit back on the exam table so he could get a better look at her cold sore.

After getting a little more information and jotting down some notes, Charlie stepped out to get Dave. They discussed treatment options for cold sores and debated the pros and cons of taking oral medication versus topical medication for episodic flare-ups, and they discussed long-term treatment options for suppression. As always, Dave suggested Charlie research the topic further and report back later.

Dave asked Charlie to see their next patient while he spoke with Ms. Robertson. He said he needed to discuss some clinic business with her.

Charlie thought about telling him about her grandson's pill bottle, but as they went their separate ways, he decided to let her do the talking.

ASSIGNMENT

Come up with a foreground (PICO) question based on this case. Find a study that answers your question, and appraise it for its Validity, Importance, and Usefulness. Use the worksheet in the appendix, and write a brief summary of the study, why you feel it answers your question adequately, and whether the study was valid, important, and useful in this case. What are some of the pros and cons of the study, and how will it impact the patient's care? What would you do after researching this question if you were the PA caring for this patient?

. . .

For the last appointment of the day, Charlie saw Curtis Lobo, a local Munising man who enjoyed hiking the trails often. He was in the office because he had noticed a rash on his abdomen that looked suspiciously like a target rash. He was there to have it looked at and get antibiotics if it was diagnosed as Lyme disease.

Curtis J. Lobo and the Case of Lyme Disease

Friday, June 5

4:45 PM

Patient: Curtis J. Lobo

Age: 57

"Good afternoon, Curtis. My name's Charlie, and I'm a PA student working with Dave. Dawn tells me you have a rash that you think is from a tick bite?" Charlie asked while greeting Curtis in room three.

"Yeah, well, ya know. I like to make things easy for ya," he replied. He lifted his shirt and showed Charlie a circular red rash about four inches wide by three inches tall with a dark red center and outer ring. The area between the center and the outer ring was faded a bit. It certainly looked like erythema migrans to Charlie.

"Did you see a tick? Or was the rash there and the tick already gone?" Charlie asked.

"Yeah, there was a tick there. I took 'em off myself. He was a fat little bugger. That was about a week ago. The rash showed up today. It's Lyme, isn't it?"

"Yup. Sure looks that way to me. Of course, Dave will have to confirm, but we'll likely have to give you an antibiotic. Are you allergic to any antibiotics?" Charlie asked.

"No. Not that I know of."

"Great. Dave will probably put you on some doxycycline. You'll need to take all of it. Don't stop early."

"Should I be worried about Lyme Disease?" Curtis asked.

"I'll let Dave answer that one for you. Let me step out and get him, and we'll get you taken care of."

In the hall, Dave and Charlie discussed Lyme disease and treatment options. They discussed symptoms to watch for that may indicate disseminated Lyme disease and ways to prevent getting Lyme disease.

They returned to the room together, and Charlie relayed the information they had just discussed to Mr. Lobo while Dave took a picture of the rash for the chart.

. . .

In Dave's office after the visit was over, Dave and Charlie discussed more treatment options for Lyme disease. They talked about prophylactic treatments, different antibiotic options, and results of studies demonstrating effective treatments. Dave asked Charlie to look into this for a PICO question or two that they'd discuss further in the morning. He had something specific to do and wanted to be out of the office on time tonight. Charlie didn't mind because he was scheduled to be somewhere as well, but he didn't tell Dave this. Some things, he felt, were told on a need-to-know basis, and at this point, where he was going tonight wasn't anything he was ready to discuss. Even though the topic of dinner would be about Dave.

ASSIGNMENT

Come up with a foreground (PICO) question based on this case. Find a study that answers your question, and appraise it for its Validity, Importance, and Usefulness. Use the worksheet in the appendix, and write a brief summary of the study, why you feel it answers your question adequately, and whether the study was valid, important, and useful in this case. What are some of the pros and cons of the study, and how will it impact the patient's care? What would you do after researching this question if you were the PA caring for this patient?

* * *

After they finished charting on the last few patients, Charlie and Dave began packing up their things in silence. Dave seemed agitated and in a hurry to get out of the office. Charlie wasn't upset or agitated, but lost in thought. He had had an odd day so far. He'd started his day overhearing a strange conversation at the campsite on Grand Island, but this paled in comparison to Jason Varney's startling reveal.

* * *

A Dinner Meeting

Ordinarily Charlie would have hiked into town for dinner, but this night he decided he'd drive. Between last night's campout and this afternoon's revelations, he didn't want to enter the woods. He had never been scared or spooked in the woods before, but now he felt uneasy about the prospect of hiking into town. Somewhere out there in the woods was a bad man who was up to no good, and Charlie didn't want anything to do with him. He wanted to ask Dave more about his suspicions, but after talking with Officer Varney, he wasn't sure Dave could be trusted either. What he needed was a burger and a beer, and he had neither at the campground.

As he drove to dinner, Charlie contemplated stopping for a beer at the American Legion but thought better of it. There were too many things at the Legion connected to his conversation with Officer Varney, and he didn't want to accidentally run into Dave or someone else there. Up North Burgers was the best place around to get burgers, at least according to Dawn, so Charlie had agreed to meet Officer Varney there. He had revealed to Charlie that he was actually an agent from DEA sent to the area to investigate Dave and the office for drug trafficking. Charlie was still in shock. He took pride in his ability to read people, and yet he never saw this coming. Charlie had suggested meeting him at Up North Burgers to discuss this further because he had reasons to believe Dave was not involved. Officer Varney wanted to know everything Charlie knew, or thought he knew. *I should have stopped for that beer,* Charlie thought as he walked in the front door of the burger joint.

Jason Varney was seated in a booth in the back and waved him over.

"Thank you for coming to talk with me," Jason said, motioning Charlie to take a seat across from him.

"Yeah. Sure. I just want you to get a chance to hear what I have to say about Dave and what he's doing. I think you've got the wrong guy."

"Not a chance. I've got it on good authority that prescriptions for narcotics are flying out of that office. He's a regular candy man, unless you know something I should know."

"Oh, come on. He shot you down when you tried to get Norco. Plus, I don't even think he has prescribed a narcotic yet this week. I just don't see it." Charlie ordered a cheeseburger and started filling Jason in as to what he had seen and heard.

"So you think there's an outside party responsible, and maybe his nurse Dawn is involved?" Jason asked.

"Well, I've seen her making suspicious exchanges with a large man, who I think might be Joseph Murphy's brother. I'm not sure."

"I'd need to be sure. Could you pick him out in a lineup? Did you take any pictures?"

"Pictures? Who do you think I am? A cop or a spy or something? I'm a PA student on rotation. The guy was big, but that's all I could really remember. I wasn't very close to see his face clearly. But if you're thinking the campsite with the stacked stones and beer cans hanging is related, it could be his brother as he is one of the only people around here who do that sort of thing."

"All right." Jason ran his hand through his hair. "Let me think this over tonight. I'll swing by the office tomorrow under the pretense that I need to have you look at the rash. If I need you for anything, I'll let you know tomorrow. The office is open in the morning, right?"

"Yeah, we open at 9 a.m."

"Okay then, I'll be there shortly after you open." Jason stood and paid the tab. "Burger's on me." He walked out without looking back.

Charlie looked at his half-eaten cheeseburger and threw his napkin over it. He'd lost his appetite.

CHAPTER 6

Saturday

Inviting Trouble

Saturday morning came with Charlie waking in a panic. He quickly reached for his phone, only to find it was 6 a.m. He'd been dreaming that he overslept and Dave had been arrested first thing that morning. The office wouldn't open for three more hours. *Thank God it was only a dream*, he thought. He tried falling back to sleep but found it difficult with his thoughts racing. He knew in his heart that Dave was innocent, and he wanted to believe that his friend Joseph was as well. He wasn't so sure about Dawn, and he had strong suspicions about Joseph's brother, if his brother was in fact actually back in town. His thoughts wandered to pondering Dave's whereabouts the previous night. Dave had spent a good deal of time this week counseling Ryan, the young man they took kayaking Thursday and Friday, and he wondered whether he was doing the same last night or if he had gone looking for Joseph's brother.

Charlie decided that if he could get the dealer to reveal himself while Officer Varney was at the office, he might be able to clear Dave in the process. But the only way he could think to get the dealer near Varney was to suggest he would buy drugs and ask for them to be delivered while Varney was there.

Charlie got dressed and headed over to the campground office. He knocked on the window, startling the young man in his twenties who worked there.

"Hey, man. You happen to know how I can get my hands on some Norco?" Charlie asked.

. . .

When Charlie got to the office, Dave's Jeep wasn't there, but Dawn's truck was. She was unlocking the front door and smiled when Charlie approached.

"Good morning, Charlie."

"Morning, Dawn. You're pretty chipper for a Saturday morning."

"We're only open for three hours on Saturday, so it's not so bad."

Charlie noticed Jason Varney standing by a tree across the street. He ambled over and met them at the front door after Dawn flipped on the neon open sign in the door's window.

"We're not quite ready for patients yet, Mr. Varney, but if you want to wait in the lobby, you can," Dawn said as she busied herself with items at the front desk.

"I can see him now and have Dave go in to see him when he gets here. It would get Mr. Varney in and out faster. All he needs is a wound check anyway," Charlie offered. "The room doesn't even need to be prepped. Just a quick peek."

"All right. Then go ahead and use room two," Dawn suggested.

Charlie gestured for Jason to enter room two and followed him in. Now would be a good time to divulge his plan to catch the real dealer and stall him on arresting Dave.

• • •

Dave arrived a few minutes later. He wasn't alone. A young man entered the front door just behind him. He looked rough. He was wearing a hoodie that obscured his face. He was fidgeting and seemed to be focused on his shoes, as if trying to go unnoticed.

"Good morning, Dawn," Dave said as he entered the lobby. "Can we get Mr. Zeller here in a room? He's been through an awful lot and could use some rest. I'll be in to talk to him in a moment. Is Charlie here yet?"

"He's already in room two with Mr. Varney for his burn recheck. He should be out soon."

Dave nodded in approval. "Good. I'll head in and see Mr. Zeller after I drop some stuff off in the office. Have Charlie wait there when he's done with Mr. Varney. I'll go in to see the wound check after I'm done with Mr. Zeller."

• • •

Sean Zeller's Headache

Saturday, June 6

9:10 AM

Patient: Sean Zeller

Age: 23

When Dave entered the room, Sean was sitting on the floor against the wall in the back corner. His knees were brought up to his chest and his head was buried in his arms that wrapped around his knees. He looked exactly as he had when he was found earlier that morning. He looked scared. Dave had been out with Joseph looking for Able, Joseph's brother. They had gone to a home where Able was known to stay in the past and found it mostly deserted. In the bedroom they heard muffled sobs and were surprised to find Sean in the closet, hiding under some clothes. When they finally coaxed him out of the closet, they found him shivering in a dirty T-shirt and jeans. He looked strung out and was noticeably high. Joseph recognized Sean as one of the blackjack dealers at the casino in Christmas. Sean was in no condition to give them any information. They decided they'd better get some fluids in him and keep him safe. That was three hours earlier. They had watched him doze on and off for hours, and when he finally was alert enough to talk, he started vomiting. Joseph vowed to continue the search without Dave, and Dave decided to bring Sean to the office to keep him safe and be sure he didn't overdose. He had no idea how much or what he had taken. He suspected an opioid.

Dave sat at the small table in the room and looked at him. Sean must have felt Dave's eyes on him because he slowly lifted his head and looked back.

"Good morning, Sean. Welcome back to the land of the living."

Sean groaned and returned to his default position, with his head down, perched on his bent knees and nest of arms.

"Can you tell me what you took last night? How much did you take? Don't worry; I'm not a cop. I'm here to help you."

He looked up again and regarded Dave for a full minute before answering. "Oxycodone."

"How many?"

"I don't really remember. Six maybe?"

"Did you get them from Able?" Dave asked.

With his head buried again in his arms, he replied with a muffled yes.

"Why were you hiding when we found you?"

Still muffled he replied, "I took some of his stuff without his knowledge. He's a rough dude. I thought you were him returning, so I hid."

"How long have you been using?"

Sean finally lifted his head and leaned back against the wall with his hands on the floor at his side. He sighed and replied, "Look, I know you mean well, but I don't need any of your help. I'm fine. I just took too much last night. That's all." He closed his eyes and sighed again. "Okay. So I've got this headache. You could give me something for that, I guess, if you really think you need to help me."

Dave could see that he was sweaty and had goose bumps on his arms. He was sniffling as well. "Sure. I can do that," he replied. Dave got up to leave when Sean stopped him.

"Hey. So I get migraines a lot. I've had headaches like this before after running out of stuff, and I've found that Norco does the best for my migraines. Any chance I can get some Norco for it?"

"Not a chance," Dave said as he left the room.

* * *

Dave found Charlie in the office waiting for him and filled him in on the situation with Sean. They discussed opioid withdrawal, headache management, and migraine management.

ASSIGNMENT

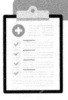

Come up with a foreground (PICO) question based on this case. Find a study that answers your question, and appraise it for its Validity, Importance, and Usefulness. Use the worksheet in the appendix, and write a brief summary of the study, why you feel it answers your question adequately, and whether the study was valid, important, and useful in this case. What are some of the pros and cons of the study, and how will it impact the patient's care? What would you do after researching this question if you were the PA caring for this patient?

• • •

Mike DeGrow and the Case of Stones

Saturday, June 6

10:30 AM

Patient: Mike DeGrow

Age: 56

After checking on Sean in room one, Dave and Charlie saw the next patient in room three, Mr. Mike DeGrow. Dawn had given them the rundown on Mr. DeGrow before they entered the room. Apparently, he awoke with severe pain in the right side of his ribs around six o'clock this morning. The pain was so severe that it made him nauseated. He was vomiting into a garbage pail now in the room. He had a low-grade fever, and his blood pressure was slightly elevated. When Charlie entered the room to see him, Mr. DeGrow looked extremely uncomfortable. He was in the fetal position on the table, cradling the garbage pail like it was his most-prized possession.

Charlie whispered to Dave, "Rough morning for patients today, heh?"

Dave nodded. "Yup."

"Good morning, Mr. DeGrow. I'm Dave Harrington, a PA here at the office, and this is Charlie. He's a PA student working with me. Dawn tells me your back hurts pretty badly. When did this start?"

Grimacing and taking quick, sharp breaths, Mike did his best to look composed as he replied. "It woke me up around six o'clock."

"On a scale from zero to ten, how would you rate your pain this morning," asked Charlie.

"Right now? A ten. It lightens up occasionally to a seven or so, but it's a ten now for sure," Mike replied. As if on cue, he vomited into the garbage pail.

"Does the pain have any relation to eating?" Charlie asked.

"No, I haven't eaten anything today. I've got no appetite," Mike replied.

"Noticed any blood in the urine, or pain with urination?" asked Dave.

"I don't know about blood, but my urine was dark this morning."

"You think you could leave us a urine sample this morning?" Dave asked. "Maybe."

Dave walked up to Mr. DeGrow and listened to his heart and lungs, tapped on his kidneys, with the right side causing some discomfort, and had him lie down to examine his abdomen. His right upper quadrant was tender, but he had a negative Murphy's sign.

"Well, if the urine sample agrees with me, I'd say you likely have a kidney stone, Mr. DeGrow. Let me talk this over with Charlie, and I'll send Dawn in to give you something for your nausea and pain. We'll be right back.

ASSIGNMENT

Come up with a foreground (PICO) question based on this case. Find a study that answers your question, and appraise it for its Validity, Importance, and Usefulness. Use the worksheet in the appendix, and write a brief summary of the study, why you feel it answers your question adequately, and whether the study was valid, important, and useful in this case. What are some of the pros and cons of the study, and how will it impact the patient's care? What would you do after researching this question if you were the PA caring for this patient?

• • •

The last patient of the morning was Ryan Perkins. Charlie recognized Ryan from the kayaking outing Thursday night and forgot that he had said he was coming in today for a follow-up. Suddenly, his plan to have Jason Varney apprehend the suspected drug dealer at the office seemed like a bad idea. If he remembered correctly, Ryan had said he would kill the man who sold Mandy her drugs if he had a chance. Charlie's stomach knotted.

Ryan Perkins and Managing Grief

Saturday, June 6

11:30 AM

Patient: Ryan Perkins

Age: 28

"Welcome back, Ryan," Dave greeted him as they entered the room. He gave Ryan a hug before they both sat down.

Charlie stood uneasily against the door, trying to think of a way to get Ryan out of the office before things got interesting.

"How did yesterday go after getting home from ecotherapy?" Dave asked.

"Good. I got home, took a shower, and practiced my meditation. I slept well for the first time in weeks last night. I think it really helped."

"Have you considered what we talked about? Have you considered Narcotics Anonymous?" Dave asked.

"Yeah. I think I'll check it out, but maybe after a week or so. It's still too raw right now."

"What about meds? Would you consider taking something for the depression?" Charlie asked, hoping to speed this along. He knew Ryan really needed more counseling and Dave could provide that, but Charlie was worried that Ryan would be in the office when the drug dealer showed up. He didn't want him to get caught up in any action.

"I don't know, man. I really think I should avoid meds right now, you know? Therapy seems good to me. I really liked that ecotherapy stuff. I can see myself doing well with that."

Dave chimed in on the medication discussion. "You know, Ryan, most medications for depression and anxiety are not narcotics. They are perfectly safe to take. There are numerous types of medications available, and they aren't intended for you to take forever. They are really only tools to help you get better. Given your history of drug issues, I'd avoid narcotics. On that we are in agreement. I promise you, we will stick to what can help and not harm you."

"I've seen some people on depression meds. They turn into zombies. They aren't depressed, but they're like in a fog instead. I don't want that."

"How about this: Charlie and I will step out a minute while you think things over, and we'll come back with some info on some of the different medications available and the pros and cons of each of them. Then you can make an educated decision. Does that sound good?" Dave asked.

Charlie didn't like how this was going. Instead of getting Ryan out of here before someone else showed up, it was looking like Ryan would be here in the middle of it all.

• • •

Charlie and Dave stepped out and headed to the office to talk it over. On the way to the office, Charlie saw Jason Varney sitting in the lobby, looking annoyed. He tapped his watch and tilted his head to the side impatiently. Charlie's stomach knotted tighter.

ASSIGNMENT

Come up with a foreground (PICO) question based on this case. Find a study that answers your question, and appraise it for its Validity, Importance, and Usefulness. Use the worksheet in the appendix, and write a brief summary of the study, why you feel it answers your question adequately, and whether the study was valid, important, and useful in this case. What are some of the pros and cons of the study, and how will it impact the patient's care? What would you do after researching this question if you were the PA caring for this patient?

* * *

It All Comes Down to This

Dave and Ryan continued their conversation from the office visit as they slowly (*painfully slowly*, Charlie thought) made their way out to the lobby. Ryan was the last patient of the day, so there was no reason for Dave to cut their conversation short. As Dave saw it, there was no rush to get Ryan out the door. Charlie, on the other hand, wanted him to get out quickly. The dealer could be here at any moment, and he didn't want Ryan to be here when he arrived.

As they entered the lobby, Dave paused his conversation with Ryan when he saw Jason Varney seated by the door.

"Mr. Varney. Did we forget something this morning? Did you need something?" Dave asked.

Jason was just starting to stand when the front door opened and two large men stepped in: Joseph Murphy and an even bigger man who could only be his brother. The resemblance was striking.

"Able," Dave muttered.

"You!" yelled Ryan. He made an attempt to lunge at Able and would have gotten to him easily if Jason Varney weren't so quick. Jason stepped between Ryan and Able, who still hadn't quite registered what was going on, and tackled Ryan to the ground. He put Ryan's hands behind his back and cuffed him.

"Settle down, young man," Varney barked. "There'll be no bloodshed on my watch."

"He gave my girlfriend the fentanyl patches that killed her!" Ryan screamed. "He needs to pay!"

Able grinned and chuckled as he looked down at Ryan on the floor.

"She's the one who asked me for 'em. It ain't my fault she couldn't handle it," Able replied.

"Shut up, Able. You're not making this any better for yourself," Joseph said.

Dave, who hadn't yet moved from the spot he stood when the Murphy brothers came in the lobby, finally spoke up.

"Able, did you give that girl drugs? I thought you would have learned your lesson by doing your time," Dave said.

"A guy's gotta make money somehow, heh?" he replied, turning his gaze to Ryan, who was now seated on the floor with his hands still cuffed behind his back. "And I've always been good at what I do. Ain't that right, Mr. Perkins?"

Jason pulled Ryan up to a standing position and asked him if he could be trusted to behave. With a curt nod from Ryan, Jason removed the cuffs and walked over to Able, who was being restrained by Joseph. He placed the cuffs on Able and took him by the arm.

"Able Murphy, you are under arrest on suspicion of second-degree murder in the death of Mandy Hillard, for drug trafficking, and for breaking parole. You have the right to remain silent. Anything you say may be ..." Jason started reciting Miranda rights to Able.

Meanwhile, Ryan slowly moved closer to Joseph, Dave asked Charlie whether Jason was a cop and if he had known previously, and Dawn disappeared.

Jason had managed to get Able turned toward the door, planning to walk him out, when Ryan pulled a deer antler-handled knife from a sheath hanging on Joseph's belt. In one quick jab, Ryan buried the knife into the left side of Able's neck. As he yanked it out, bright red blood pulsed out, hitting the doorframe and quickly covering Able's shirt. Jason shot a surprised look over his shoulder to Ryan, but he wasn't quick enough to stop him from burying the knife to the hilt in Able's side. Able crumpled to the floor, fumbling at the wound in his neck as his blood-soaked shirt began to drip fresh red blood on the floor.

Jason lunged at Ryan's arm, and they both slipped in the blood that was now pooling on the floor below them. As they wrestled for the knife, Charlie stood and watched in horror, unable to move or think. Dave and Joseph went to Able and tried to apply pressure to his wounds.

"Call for an ambulance!" Dave yelled out to Dawn.

Dawn, who had been mysteriously absent for the carnage, came out of the back office with a fire extinguisher. She approached the scuffling men on the floor, raised the fire extinguisher over her head, and came down hard, connecting with the back of Ryan's head. She repeated the motion, connecting with Jason's head in the same manner. They both crumpled to the floor unconscious. Dave and Joseph looked up with disbelief to see Dawn standing there with a backpack on her back and a bloody fire extinguisher in her hands.

"Is he going to die?" she asked, gesturing with the fire extinguisher to Able.

"He will if he doesn't get an ambulance soon," replied Dave.

"So why don't we put that down and call for one!" added Joseph.

"Nah, I think we'd all be better off if he just died," she replied. She tossed the fire extinguisher to Charlie, bringing him out of his daze, and stepped over the unconscious men and around Able. Then she walked outside and started running in the direction of the Pipeline trailhead.

Charlie, now fully alert and aware for the first time since the bloodshed began, put the fire extinguisher down and ran to the phone to call for help.

A few minutes later the sound of sirens could be heard coming their way. Ryan and Jason had begun to stir but were only moaning. Charlie was helping Dave and Joseph care for Able's wounds. He was worried. He had never seen so much blood.

New Beginnings

One Year Later

Charlie arrived to work a full thirty minutes early. He wanted to check out the view of Grand Island from the back patio of the clinic before starting the day and the tourism season. He unlocked the front door and put his things in the back office. The office looked almost exactly like it had when he first arrived the previous summer. The only noticeable changes were some freshly painted walls and his name on the desk in place of Dave Harrington's.

The bell over the front door jingled.

"Good morning, Mr. Brinker!" a cheerful voice called out from the waiting room.

Charlie smiled. "Good morning, Mrs. Swienhart!" he called back. It was nice to hear Carol Swienhart's voice. The kind old nurse who had filled in last summer for Dawn had been hired full-time this summer. It was good to have a seasoned veteran on board during his first summer working alone in a clinic. Dawn was still missing, and the owner of the clinic wasn't ever going to hire her back anyway.

After Ryan had recovered enough to talk to detectives, it had come out that Dawn was actually Ryan's cousin and she had pretended to be a nurse and falsified records to deceive the owner of the clinic. Her role was to steal blank prescription pads from the office and give them to Ryan through Able as a middleman. Able had used some of the prescriptions to fill fentanyl without Ryan's blessing or knowledge and had given some to Mandy, leading to her overdose. Ryan was the drug dealer in control of all the narcotics in Munising, and Dawn was an accomplice. Able had tried to one-up him, and it backfired. When Able looked to be on his way to meet his maker, Dawn saw an opportunity to make a run for it and took it.

Jason and Ryan survived their head injuries, and Able fought admirably before losing his battle in the ICU in Marquette. Joseph stayed in Marquette after his brother's passing and started taking classes at Northern Michigan University to be a counselor. Charlie thought he would be a great counselor in ecotherapy. Dave left the clinic after the trial ended and started a rehab clinic with a few other PAs and doctors in Munising.

"Looks like we'll be hitting the ground running this season, Mr. Brinker," Carol said, poking her head in the door of the back office.

"Please, just call me Charlie."

"We've already got some patients, Charlie. You're needed in room one."

When Charlie opened the door to room one, he was greeted by a group of young Boy Scouts, and he couldn't help but smile.

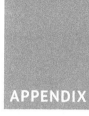

Research Article Appraisal Worksheet

PICO question:

_____

_____

Article being reviewed:

_____

_____

Are the results of the study VALID?

1. Were the patients in the study randomized?
2. Was the randomization concealed?
3. How long was the follow-up? Was it complete?
4. Was there blinding used?
5. Were the groups treated the same?

If the results of the study are VALID, are they also IMPORTANT?

1. What is the 95% Confidence Interval (95% CI)?
2. What is the number needed to treat/harm (NNT or NNH)?

If the results are deemed VALID and IMPORTANT, can you apply them to the patient in question?

1. Is the case patient similar to the patients in the study?

2. Is the intervention/treatment/diagnostic test being studied feasible in the setting of the case?

3. What are the potential benefits or harms of implementing this intervention/treatment/diagnostic test?

4. Do you know the patient's values/preferences, and does this intervention/treatment/diagnostic test have any conflict with the values/preferences of the case patient?

References

Agius, A.M., J.M. Pickles, and K.L. Burch. 1992. "A Prospective Study of Otitis Externa." *Clin Otolaryngol Allied Sci* 17 (2): 150–54.

Alshryda, S., A. Shah, S. Odak, J. Al-Shryda, B. Ilango, and S.R. Murali. 2012. "Acute Fractures of the Scaphoid Bone: Systematic Review and Meta-Analysis." *Surgeon* 10 (4): 218–29.

Bhaumik, S., R. Kirubakaran, and S. Chaudhuri. 2019. "Primary Closure Versus Delayed or No Closure for Traumatic Wounds Due to Mammalian Bite." *Cochrane Database of Systematic Reviews* 12 (12).

Bitter, C.C. and T.B. Erickson. 2016. "Management of Burn Injuries in the Wilderness: Lessons from Low-Resource Settings." *Wilderness Environ Med* 27 (4): 519–25.

Borghi, C. and M. Veronesi. 2019. "Cough and ACE Inhibitors: The Truth Beyond Placebo." *Clinical Pharmacology Therapy* 105 (3): 550–52.

Choi, H.K., K. Atkinson, E.W. Karlson, W. Willette, and G. Curhan. 2004. "Alcohol Intake and Risk of Incident Gout in Men: a Prospective Study." *Lancet* 363 (9417): 1277–81.

Deshpande, A., V. Pasupuleti, P. Thota, C. Pant, D.D. Rolston, T.J. Sferra, et al. 2013. "Community-Associated Clostridium Difficile Infection and Antibiotics: a Meta-Analysis." *Journal of Antimicrob Chemother* 68 (9): 1951–61.

Vinik, A.I., M.L. Nevoret, C. Casellini, and H. Parson. 2013. "Diabetic Neuropathy." *Endocrinol Metab Clin North Am.* 42 (4): 747–87.